It's Not My Head, It's My Hormones

How to tame your hormones
and feel like yourself again

DR MARION GLUCK

First published in Great Britain in 2019 by Orion Spring
an imprint of The Orion Publishing Group Ltd
Carmelite House, 50 Victoria Embankment
London EC4Y 0DZ

An Hachette UK Company

5 7 9 10 8 6 4

Every effort has been made to ensure that the information in the book
is accurate. The information in this book may not be applicable in each
individual case so it is advised that professional medical advice is obtained
for specific health matters and before changing any medication or dosage.
Neither the publisher nor author accepts any legal responsibility for any
personal injury or other damage or loss arising from the use of the
information in this book. In addition, if you are concerned about
your diet or exercise regime and wish to change them, you
should consult a health practitioner first.

A CIP catalogue record for this book is
available from the British Library.

ISBN (Trade paperback) 978 1 4091 7856 9
ISBN (eBook) 978 1 4091 7857 6

Printed and bound in Great Britian by Clays Ltd, Elcograf, S.p.A

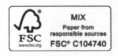

MIX
Paper from
responsible sources
FSC® C104740

ORION
SPRING

www.orionbooks.co.uk

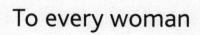

To every woman

CONTENTS

● ● ● ●

INTRODUCTION

● ● ● ●

Hormones are finally getting the attention they deserve. They are of great importance to our health and well-being. They provide the background music to all women's lives.

Our sex hormones come on-stream at puberty, when oestrogen in particular sculpts lips, breasts and the extra fat beneath the skin. This is when their production normally settles into a monthly rhythm that switches between oestrogen and progesterone and the moods that flow with them. Hormones also orchestrate the far larger changes – physical and emotional – that accompany pregnancy and childbirth. In our middle age their production begins to fall off, and as we head into menopause, their music gradually fades.

Menopause is best known as 'the change', a time of hormonal transformation and physical and mental adjustment. But women are hormonal beings all through their lives, and puberty, pregnancy and perimenopause may also be times of hormonal upheaval and imbalance. This book will talk about the journey of how hormones change throughout your life and how they impact on your mind as well as your body. Often the years in the run-up to menopause can be the most challenging time in a woman's life, and I will talk about this as the book goes on.

It is not unusual for some women at menopause to be ashamed

to find themselves without their sex hormones and thus feel redundant as sexual, attractive and loving beings. They may feel their 'use-by date' has been reached and that they are no longer sexually wanted or needed.

This book is here to help women (and men) understand that they are not losing their mind or going crazy. Hormones have a profound impact on the way we feel, think and act.

It's about time we educated ourselves on the effects of our hormones and their relationship to our body and our brain chemistry so we can embrace these 'sparks' of life. It's about time we listened to these chemical messengers and understood what they are saying.

Today there is a growing awareness of mental health issues and their consequences. The diagnosis of depression and the use of antidepressants is on the rise. Why is this so? Why are one in four people suffering? Awareness is great and important but there is still not enough understanding about possible causes and factors contributing to this mental health epidemic, such as our hormonal health, lifestyle and stressors.

My hope is that through this book, hormones and their effect on brain chemistry will be simplified and demystified for you; that you will understand how hormones affect you and your moods and actions as an individual; how science, politics and commercial interests have limited your options; and how your choice of how you manage your hormones can help you take control of your physical and mental well-being.

In 2010 I wrote *It Must Be My Hormones*. I wanted women to know and understand the impact hormones have on their physical welfare. I felt it was important to demystify bio-identical hormones, which are identical to our own naturally occurring hormones and are derived from plant or 'phyto' extracts, specifically found in soy and yams. This differentiates them from the synthetic hormones used in conventional hormone replacement therapy (HRT), which have a different molecular structure to body-identical (bio-identical) hormones. Synthetic hormones are manmade drugs which act as hormones but can have severe side effects compared to the hormones our body produces naturally.

I wanted to take the fear factor out of hormone therapy. But there is still much left unsaid and misunderstood. This is why I have decided to write about the connections between mind, mood and hormones.

Today we have far greater knowledge of the various ways the smooth working of our hormones can become disrupted by pollutants or plastics in our environment and by our lifestyle – especially diet and stress. Yet we still face an ocean of confusion when hormonal levels drop, or their rhythms fall out of sync. There is little consensus in the medical world and even less on the internet about the best way to handle such changes. In fact, hormone-related complaints are more prevalent today than when I first started practising medicine over thirty years ago.

My journey

I have several decades of experience of helping and learning from my patients and I know I can positively affect their lives when they have despaired of finding a solution to problems such as experiencing a dangerous hormonal high or running on empty.

What surprised me, even as a young doctor practising in Australia, was just how limited the understanding and treatment options were that regular doctors could offer when a patient's rhythms became discordant and their emotions erratic. We live with tides that ebb and flow through our bodies with the potential to make us feel sexy, loving, furious and sad, most notably in puberty, during pregnancy and around the menopause, yet the most widely used treatment for menopause was a standard dose of just two synthetic hormones, Premarin and Provera. They are substitutes for only oestrogen and progesterone, despite our ovaries and adrenal glands producing several other sex hormones (oestradiol, oestriol, testosterone and DHEA) that are all major hormonal players.

My approach to medicine was always considered 'outside of the box' even in my early days, when I cultivated an open mind to alternative therapies. I was a child of the sixties, and women's liberation was bursting onto the scene. Women and their well-being became my *raison d'être*. I wanted to empower women, through knowledge, to take responsibility for their own health. The subject of the effects of our own hormones on our bodies, and hormone treatment – hormonal contraception and HRT – was becoming better known amongst the general public and medical professionals. But what did this mean; what kind of hormones and what kind of treatment was going to work for my patients?

I quickly realised that many doctors and the medical industry as a whole seemed only interested in treating symptoms. We were taught to name a disease by diagnosing it, then treat it with either medicine or surgery. The disease or problem was detached from the person who had it. The individual patient was not of particular interest. We had a job to do and were not expected to think too much about what had caused a disease; only to treat what we could diagnose. This has evolved into the world of medicine we see today, where targets and budgets and ticking boxes to prove results seem more important than the well-being of those caught up in the system.

This seemed to me to be a medical cul-de-sac, and I managed

to find a way to avoid it by adopting an approach to patients with hormonal issues that focused on their distinctive individual needs, but which was also firmly scientifically based. Listening to patients and building a rapport with them has been my main focus from the very beginning. The result was that my practice grew. Patients would come into the clinic not understanding what was happening and why they were feeling unlike themselves. They were anxious and insecure, and when I could explain what was happening to them in this period of their life, they felt a great sense of relief. After all, hormonal change is normal and should be addressed and remedied in a natural way. Among the patients I was able to help were some who had spent years going around in ineffective circles with mainstream medicine looking for understanding and answers.

At the heart of my approach was the use of a type of hormone known as bio-identical, which means that their chemical make-up is exactly the same as the natural hormones your body produces. It may come as a surprise to learn that the oestrogen and progesterone you get in the birth control pill or in HRT are different to those you make naturally. Your doctor is very unlikely to tell you this. I believe that if you are replacing something in a system as complex and sophisticated as the human body, it makes sense to use a formula that has evolved over millions of years, rather than a recipe recently cooked up in a lab. There is now lots of evidence, which I cover later, that the synthetic or 'fake' hormones can cause damaging side effects that you don't get with bio-identical hormones.

In this book, when I write about hormones, I am writing about either those hormones we produce naturally as part of our own biological processes, or those classed as 'bio-identical', which can be used to supplement or replace our own naturally occurring hormones as they decline over time. These bio-identical hormones, derived from plant extracts, can replicate the molecular structure of our own naturally produced hormones. I am an advocate of this approach because in my view it makes sense to replace like with like and follow what nature intended.

This is what built my reputation as a pioneer and firebrand in the world of bio-identical hormone replacement therapy (BHRT). I brought a new approach to women's health – and indeed men's too – with BHRT and individualised care. At the time it was a controversial treatment, but today it has become more mainstream, as there is an unsatisfied demand for 'common sense' medicine that works and is safe.

A great source of inspiration to me was one of my heroines, Dr Katharina Dalton, who had been the pioneer of bio-identical hormone therapy in London in the 1960s and understood women and their psyches. Like me, she had swum against the tide of her times, keeping faith in her own convictions, such as the link between hormones and depression, and proving her theories with meticulous research.

She linked mental health to hormone fluctuations and introduced natural progesterone therapy, with great success, to women worldwide. She coined the phrase premenstrual syndrome (PMS) and in 1957 started the world's first PMS clinic at University College Hospital in London, where for forty years she was a beacon of hope for thousands of women.

Like Dalton, I also questioned and thought about what made us tick as human beings. What is behaviour and what is mood? What is it that actually affects and influences our physiology so that we respond mentally and physically the way we do? Why are some people placid and calm and others can go into a sudden rage for no apparent reason?

Introduction

When I arrived in the UK in 2006, I found a dynamic society bubbling with energy and ideas, and individuals with a growing interest in understanding their own health and taking control of their futures. I was encouraged by this environment to set up my own clinic in central London and have never looked back. The Marion Gluck Clinic is the first dedicated women's health clinic in the UK specialising in the bespoke treatment of hormonal imbalances with bio-identical hormones.

I love London as it has enabled me to work in the way I believe medicine should be practised, to take the time to listen to my patients, understand their situations and respect each individual. The overwhelmingly positive response from my patients, confirming their appreciation of personalised medicine, continues to inspire me.

By the time my clinic was up and running, it had become clear that to provide a complete individual service to patients I needed a compounding pharmacy – a pharmacy specialising in personalised medications – to produce the tailor-made combinations of hormones they required. Patients may benefit from different doses of the main hormones, progesterone and oestrogen, along with other hormones that interact with them: testosterone, important for the libido, DHEA for adrenals, and the thyroid hormones for energy and metabolism. A bio-identical prescription to help with the menopause is far more sophisticated and complex than the two fixed doses in a regular HRT tablet. This is bespoke hormone therapy for each patient

Mainstream doctors have long criticised the use of bio-identical hormones on two grounds: that they lack evidence of safety and effectiveness, and that the use of compounding pharmacies is unsafe and could result in patients getting contaminated preparations in the wrong dose. Both criticisms are based on a lack of understanding. Later we will look at evidence for the greater effectiveness of bio-identicals, while the concern about compounding pharmacies ignores the fact that all major hospitals have such a pharmacy, and all are strictly regulated. Basically, I was practising old-fashioned medicine. In the 1930s and 1940s, approximately 60 per cent of all medications were compounded, but by the 1960s, mass-produced tablets had become the norm.

While tablets are very inflexible, a compounding system can provide not only unique combinations, but also different delivery systems, such as a lozenge that can be absorbed under the tongue or a cream to go on the skin. The Marion Gluck Clinic is now no longer a 'one-man band' but a successful international organisation employing a group of dedicated doctors.

However, we will never lose sight of the individual as our focal point, and our mission is to transform lives through an innovative, ethical and compassionate approach to treatment that is tailor-made to each patient.

So I come full circle back to the root of my interest: trying to understand what makes us 'tick' and understanding hormones and their role in affecting every function in our body and mind.

Our hormones are our friends – we should not fear them but embrace them. They are the initiators of our behaviour, our mood, our emotions and our actions. You will soon become aquainted with these powerful hormones that rule our lives, and you will learn how to manage them in the way nature intended.

I will explore and explain how and why hormones affect our mind, and how our mind affects our mood, and how our mood affects our behaviour, and how our behaviour in its own turn affects our mind. You will appreciate why we act, feel and think the way we do in the different phases of our lives and become familiar with the delicate balance between hormones and brain chemistry. This book is about us all, and specifically, it's about you. It is to help you to know and understand yourself better.

By reading it, I hope you will be given the tools to appreciate and understand yourself, your actions and reactions. When at times you may feel anxious or sad, or just not like yourself, you will be able to recognise how your hormones are affecting your life. With this new-found wisdom will come an understanding of the moods and feelings you experience. You will realise that, in spite of your best efforts, it is not always you who is in control; it can be your hormones 'going haywire'. Understanding yourself will help you help yourself.

Ultimately, without this understanding we risk being undermined by our own minds and bodies, but with it we may have a winning hand. I will keep shouting it from the rooftops, as I have done throughout my professional life. We have nothing to be afraid of. Hormones are a girl's (and man's) best friend!

CHAPTER ONE
THE HORMONE PUZZLE

• • • •

The word hormone comes from the Greek verb *ormào* (ὁρμάω), which means 'to impel or set in motion' or 'to arouse or excite'. Hormones are part of a highly complex interconnected network of chemical controllers and messengers that influence our thoughts, feelings and behaviour. They provide us with energy and vitality, but they can also plunge us into gloom and despair.

They play a leading role in whom we love and whom we don't. Their proper functioning is vital for our health; for strong bones, shiny hair and glowing skin. They are also essential for good digestion and how well we absorb our food. They allow us to stay a healthy weight, sleep well and handle stress effectively, and they play a central role in our brains.

Hormones also help us to recognise danger and to respond to it rapidly and effectively. That is why they can change when we are stressed. They also make us into the women and men we are and contribute to every function of our body, physical and mental. We cannot live without hormones.

In my clinic I often see women who have suddenly found themselves plunged into an emotional state that they don't recognise and are looking for help. These cases show very vividly just how much hormones affect how we think and feel on a day-to-day basis, and how you may not realise just what they have been doing for you until they are gone.

CASE STUDY: SALLY

Sally came to see me feeling desperate. For some months she had been in a terrible state, her emotions all over the place. It had all begun very suddenly. One morning she had woken up with a knot in her stomach and a sense of impending doom. On the way home after dropping the children at school, she had had a panic attack, overcome by a fear that something awful might be happening to her. The next morning she woke again with this sensation in her stomach and mild anxiety. She had no idea why this was happening, and when her husband came home, she burst into tears for no apparent reason and couldn't stop crying.

After that, she woke up every morning plagued by feelings of fear and worry, which seemed to have no connection with what was happening in her life. She began to isolate herself, stopping socialising and going to the gym. Eventually she went to see her GP and told him that she no longer 'felt like herself' and was constantly worried that something would happen to her family. She said she couldn't explain why this was so but hoped that he could tell her what was happening. He quickly diagnosed her with anxiety and depression and prescribed antidepressants. But Sally insisted she was not depressed; she had no reason to feel this way as nothing had changed in her life. She came to see me because she wanted to know what was going on.

I ran some tests and found that something had indeed changed in her life. She was forty-four years of age and her menopause was beginning – she was perimenopausal. The levels of various hormones in her body were fluctuating and it was this that was causing her distressing symptoms. The tests showed she had low levels of oestrogen and virtually no progesterone. For years her ovaries had triggered the release of these hormones when she ovulated (produced an egg ready to be fertilised) each month, but now she was no longer ovulating regularly. The combination of low oestrogen and no progesterone was causing her anxiety.

The perimenopause is probably the most challenging time in a woman's life. Her hormones can be all over the place. Periods may be scant, or flooding, or irregular. Mood swings may become the norm, fluctuating between sudden fits of anger or irritability and unprecedented desperation, uncontrollable crying and anxiety. Anything can happen. It's why many women like Sally say: 'I just don't feel like myself.'

Once this was understood, the solution was easy. A prescription of bio-identical hormones, uniquely formulated for Sally's needs, was able to mimic what should be happening naturally during a menstrual cycle, and the anxiety and mood swings cleared up.

The tragedy is what happened in her GP's surgery. Although it is no secret that women's moods become more erratic around the menopause, and that it often begins in the mid forties, doctors still rarely ask why this is happening, or what has changed in their patient's life that is causing such symptoms. Instead of diagnosing a hormonal imbalance, they diagnose depression and prescribe antidepressants, drugs that are often ineffective and come with a nasty range of side effects, including the possibility of becoming addicted.

The symptoms Sally and others might experience can be part of depression, but that doesn't mean they are suffering from clinical depression. Understanding what is going on will allow you to have a much more informed conversation about it with your doctor.

How hormones were discovered

Doctors have known about the actions of hormones for over a hundred years; they were isolated and purified in the 1930s, making hormonal treatment possible.

At the end of the nineteenth century, conventional scientific wisdom was that the messages that flashed around the body were all controlled by electric pulses in the nerves, although a few speculated that something else might be involved. Then in 1905, while experimenting on how messages arrived at a dog's pancreas, an English physiologist called Ernest Starling and his partner William Bayliss made a remarkable discovery. In a series of famous speeches to the Royal Society in London, Starling referred to 'chemical messengers, which speeding from cell to cell along the bloodstream, may coordinate the activities and growth of different parts of the body'.[1]

By all accounts Starling was at a dinner at a Cambridge college when he asked a fellow academic, who happened to be a classicist, to suggest a name for his newly identified messengers. The answer came back with the ancient Greek *ormào*, which turned into 'hormon', meaning 'movement with force'.

Interestingly, the psychiatrist and psychoanalyst Carl Jung (1875–1961) also used the word 'horme' to describe what he referred to as 'hypothetical mental energy that drives unconscious activities and instincts'.[2] Jung seems to have realised that there was a connection between mental energy, emotions and behaviour.

---

1 John Henderson, 'Ernest Starling and "Hormones": an historical commentary', *Journal of Endocrinology*, Vol. 184, Issue 1. Available at: https://joe.bioscientifica.com/view/journals/joe/184/1/1840005.xml.
2 C. G. Jung, *The Structure and Dynamics of the Psyche* (Routledge, 1970).

This is perhaps the first established link between these as yet unnamed hormones and the mind.

I find it fascinating that we have only really known about these chemicals for such a short period, yet the story of hormones goes back much further and is filled with eccentrics convinced they would find a 'magic potion' to restore vitality and youth.

The concept of invisible internal forces had its roots in ancient times. There are tales from China of older women drinking the urine of young women to stave off ageing, and stories of ancient Greeks and Romans eating animal testicles to increase their virility. Our ancient forebears believed there were hidden forces they could tap into. They were not wrong.

An early pioneer of hormone medicine, or endocrinology, was Charles-Édouard Brown-Séquard, one of the most colourful characters in nineteenth-century science, who carried out rejuvenation experiments on himself using daily injections of guinea pigs' and dogs' testicular blood and seminal fluids, which, he claimed, made him feel thirty years younger. He published the results in 1889.[3] Brown-Séquard clearly demonstrated that we cannot live without hormones, even though these mysterious chemicals had yet to be identified. His fluids became famous as a treatment for the various disorders of old age, and though controversial, his intuition about 'internal secretions' did prove to have substance. He is known as 'the father of modern endocrinology'. In the 1930s, his fluids became the basis for identifying testosterone. Scientists wanted to discover what the secret agent or chemical was that made one feel strong and energetic when the fluids were injected.

---

3   C. E. Brown-Séquard, 'Note on the effects produced on man by subcutaneous injections of a liquid obtained from the testicles of animals,' *The Lancet*, July 1889, Vol. 134, Issue 3438, pp.105–107. Available at: https://www.sciencedirect.com/science/article/pii/S0140673600641181.

Meanwhile, scientists were also trying to find the active ingredient produced by the ovaries. In 1897, an ovary extract proved to be effective for the treatment of menopausal hot flushing. Then, in 1906, ovary extracts caused monkeys to become sexually active on a regular basis. This is known as oestrus, from the Greek *oistros* (mad desire) and *gennan* (to produce), forming the basis for the word 'oestrogen'.

In the 1930s, improved techniques allowed researchers to isolate the three types of oestrogen – oestrone, oestradiol and oestriol – from the urine of pregnant women and progesterone from the placenta. By the 1940s, the preferred raw material for oestrogen was the urine of pregnant mares, which is still being used to make the artificial oestrogen Premarin (PREgnant MAre urINe!). This hormone does not have precisely the same structure as the version made in the human body. As covered in more detail in the next chapter, the version of progesterone then, and now, being used by the medical profession was also not identical to that made in the body.

Interest really stepped up in the 1950s with the development of the oral contraceptive pill (OCP). This is arguably one of the most significant developments of the whole period, with the birth control pill often listed in the top ten most important discoveries of the twentieth century. Implications for women, society, the workplace, the family and indeed every part of modern life were huge.

I feel very strongly that the development of the OCP, which gave women the ability to regulate their fertility, was a hugely empowering development. However, the physical effect of controlling fertility hormones was so significant that little research was done on the impact that it has on our mental state. In fact there had been stirrings of speculation about the emotional and mental effect of these hormones, but they were perhaps understandably eclipsed by the enormous implications of such a ground-breaking discovery for disease and illness, and how it could be harnessed to give women control over their fertility

In the twenty-first century, mental health is now a burning topic and it's time we really understood the role hormones play in undermining or improving our mood and emotions. This knowledge will be as transformative for our future as the development of the OCP was in our past.

The brain's highway: hormones and neurotransmitters

There is a profound relationship between hormones, neurotransmitters and the brain. Hormones are precision-made molecules that regulate all major bodily functions, like the cogs of a machine that assure perfect movement, or like the instruments in an orchestra that together play a beautiful harmonious symphony. When one instrument is out of tune, or a cog is stuck, it affects the whole performance; without hormone harmony, we suffer physical and mental malaise and our body and mind falter.

Why is it that we sometimes feel happy, vital and sexy and at other times angry, depressed, anxious and frustrated? How is it that some hormones actually make us feel happy or unhappy, or make us well or unwell?

We produce happiness- or feel-good-inducing brain chemicals such as dopamine, serotonin and endorphins. These brain chemicals or neurotransmitters are under the direct influence of our sex hormones, particularly oestrogen and progesterone. Hormones and neurotransmitters should act in unison, but when this delicate balance is interrupted, mood swings, anger, depression and anxiety result. Unruly and disorganised hormones, especially during perimenopause, can trigger a series of negative emotions and thoughts by disrupting neurotransmission, the messaging pathway. Science now confirms that there is a feedback loop between body and mind, and we are more prone to emotional instability if our hormones are in disarray.

All physiological and psychological actions can be attributed at some level to our hormones. Sex hormones have a profound effect on brain chemistry and how we feel. Depending on a woman's hormonal cycle, oestrogen and progesterone arouse different mood-related effects and physical functions. Mid cycle, when a woman ovulates, her oestrogen peaks and her sex drive is heightened. After ovulation, when progesterone peaks, the frenzy settles down and a sense of relaxation kicks in.

Hormones are crucial for us to feel sexy or be sexually attractive to others. Sexual attraction results from the hormones and pheromones we release in certain situations; some will turn us on, while others will turn us off!

The upside of hormones is that they can infuse in us a sense of enthusiasm, purpose and vitality. They can help us maintain a life of health and happiness with a deep satisfaction in the very fact that we are alive.

But there can also be downsides, including severe mood swings and depression when the interplay between hormones, brain chemicals and our body is disrupted or misaligned.

Because hormones are so complex and still somewhat mysterious, even doctors have felt intimidated by the intricacies of the hormone regulation system and the mind–body connection. Often they neglect to ask the necessary intimate questions, concerning, for instance, mood and the menstrual cycle, or libido, or painful intercourse, which for some patients could be difficult to discuss, especially due to cultural or religious taboos. Young girls and women are often embarrassed about the changes and sensations they are experiencing in their bodies and doctors are sometimes too timid to ask.

It can be difficult to put into words what you are experiencing, how you feel out of control, angry, depressed, overwhelmed, sad, lost, helpless or hopeless. Perhaps your libido has gone and you feel unattractive. At other times you might feel euphoric, filled with joy and love, experiencing contentment and peace, sympathy, empathy, ambition, passion, vitality and a zest for life. How can one explain these emotional and behavioural changes?

This range of emotions may strike us all at different times, with feelings brought about by circumstance, our environment, our life situation, our hormones and our brain chemistry.

Hormones misunderstood

All too often I have had perimenopausal patients come to me as a last resort after their GP has told them nothing is wrong and to 'go home and accept that you are getting older'. On the other hand, I frequently see patients who have complained to their GPs of anxiety, fatigue, insomnia or just not feeling like themselves for no apparent reason. The response is often a diagnosis of depression, especially after the patient has ticked all the right boxes on the depression questionnaire that every GP has handy on his or her desk. They may only need as few as eight questions, which all are very broad, such as: how much pleasure do you take in life? Do you feel depressed? Do you have trouble falling asleep or have little energy? The remedy is often antidepressants, anti-anxiety medication or sleeping tablets – or all three!

Here is a list of symptoms that are common to both hormonal imbalance and depression. An open-minded doctor should consider both possibilities.

- hopelessness
- apathy
- anxiety
- low mood
- lack of enthusiasm
- fatigue or low energy
- poor appetite or overeating
- lack of confidence
- lack of concentration
- restlessness
- low libido
- insomnia
- suicidal thoughts

As we saw in the case of Sally, who was moving into her menopause without realising it, changes in hormone levels can have a variety of psychological effects – anxiety, insomnia, loss of self-confidence. So how much better would it be to restore hormones to the level they were before? Given that bio-identical hormones don't disrupt the natural hormonal system already active in the brain, I believe it is time doctors became more aware of the potential of these hormones to allow patients to feel normal and well again.

So we have a sophisticated natural system for regulating our emotions, which benefits from bio-identical hormones but not artificial ones. But we have only looked at what happens in female brains.

What happens in the men we married, or our brothers, friends and fathers? Are they always on top form, or do their moods change to irritability, short-temperedness or just lack of drive and enthusiasm at different times of their lives?

Of course the same disruption happens to men, especially during their 'andropause' or male menopause, which is some-time referred to as 'the midlife crisis'. While some men take Viagra, others buy motorbikes or new sports cars or have affairs. Men with low hormonal levels (primarily testosterone) may lose their drive and enthusiasm and can also succumb to terrible mood swings, including irritability, anger or depression. They may also present their GP with their symptoms and walk out with a diagnosis of depression. A recent paper in *JAMA Psychiatry* reported on the benefits of supplementing with testosterone.[4]

The effect of sex hormones on men, specifically testosterone, isn't limited to the midlife crisis. Daily life, family, bereavement, stress, relationships can all produce some of the feelings mentioned above, such as hopelessness, anxiety, low mood and fatigue or low energy.

Nevertheless, we must not confuse 'feeling depressed' with a depressive mental health illness. The former may respond to lifestyle changes, hormone replacement or stress reduction and counselling, whereas the latter may certainly require antidepressant medication, ideally with support from psychotherapy or cognitive behavioural therapy.

All too often one is diagnosed with depression when one is sad or melancholic. This is usually due to a trauma such as bereave-

---

4   A. Walther, J. Breidenstein and R. Miller, 'Association of Testosterone Treatment with Alleviation of Depressive Symptoms in Men', *JAMA Psychiatry*. Published online 14 November 2018. Available at: doi:10.1001/jamapsychiatry.2018.2734.

ment or a lifestyle situation such as chronic stress, and is known as an exogenous depression; the cause comes from the outside and we should always treat the cause and not the symptom. Endogenous depressions, on the other hand – moods and feelings and thoughts that come from the inside – may be caused by genetic or biological factors and are often referred to as 'biologically' based.

Your GP may ask you to fill in a standard depression questionnaire with its broad generalised questions, mentioned above. Who hasn't experienced some of those symptoms to varying degrees? Does it really mean you suffer from depression, or are there other factors that may be contributing to how you feel?

You may well be prescribed antidepressants if you respond positively to some symptoms on this list, but have you been asked follow-up questions about why you are feeling this way? What are your circumstances? Has anyone in your family died? Are you under too much pressure at work? Do you have financial problems or difficult relationship issues? How long have you had some of the symptoms, and are they recurring? The list of questions and their answers is long, but they need to be taken into consideration if patients are to be properly diagnosed.

One of the ways to distinguish between hormonal imbalance and depression is to consider that very often a hormonal cause is recurrent and/or cyclical. Moods and feelings may appear at certain times of the month, especially with women. Men can also suffer from recurrent moods, especially at weekends, when they begin to relax from the stress of work and responsibility. This appears often as headache or migraine. How many men do you know who suffer from headaches at the weekend and not during the week? The reason is that under duress or stress, hormones such as cortisol are elevated and mask or protect us from the fatigue or anxiety or pain symptoms we may be experiencing. This enables us to carry on when in need.

The number of antidepressants prescribed in the UK between 2005 and 2015 has more than doubled. But is it really possible that as a society we are getting more depressed year by year?

I believe that as doctors and primary care health practitioners we should be more open-minded when considering that there may be other reasons, and solutions, for mood swings, or when a patient says, 'I just don't feel like myself anymore.' Patients, both men and women, should not be diagnosed, labelled and dismissed as suffering from depression just because they tick a few simple boxes.

Many patients are now questioning their doctors more deeply and are also becoming more proactive in their healthcare decisions. Knowledge is power, and patients want to know what is happening to them, why they feel unwell and what they can do about it.

So, in addition to the symptoms listed above, I always ask my patients if they are suffering from any of the following – some of which obviously only apply to females:

- night sweats
- hot flushes
- vaginal dryness
- incontinence
- joint aches and pains
- headaches
- dry skin
- hair loss
- memory loss
- fuzzy brain

- heart palpitations
- numbness of hands and feet
- crawling skin sensation
- crying spells
- dizziness
- shortness of breath
- anxiety
- anger
- irritability
- lack of confidence
- lack of enthusiasm

It's important for me to know as much as possible about my patients, their symptoms and their circumstances. I would hope all medical practitioners feel the same, but do challenge your doctor to consider all possibilities.

Help is on the way: the introduction of bio-identical hormones

Bio-identical hormones are identical to the naturally occurring hormones that our bodies produce. They are identical because they have the same molecular structure as our own hormones, and they are the perfect fit for the hormone receptors in our bodies. They function like our own and are the best replacement that nature can provide for our hormones. Everything else is an inferior substitute. Bio-identical hormones are essential to maintaining hormone health and mental and physical well-being in the case of hormone fluctuation or decline.

SUMMARY OF KEY POINTS

- Hormones form a chemical web that affects every part of our body as well as our thoughts and feelings.
- They can make us feel wonderful but also plunge us into anxiety and fury or depression and despair when levels change and they become unbalanced.
- One of the most common instances of hormonal imbalance is the menopause, which can be the most challenging time of a woman's life.
- Hormones and their decline are the cause of the menopausal roller coaster, yet the treatment is all too often antidepressants that do nothing to help these hormone levels.
- Scientists have known about hormones for over a hundred years. They were first used as a treatment in the 1930s.
- Many ancient cultures believed in 'forces' in the body that controlled its functions.
- In the late nineteenth century, injections of blood and fluids from animal testicles were used as an anti-ageing treatment for men.
- Oestrogen, extracted from the urine of pregnant mares, was being used as a treatment for menopause in the 1940s.
- The use of hormones to create a contraceptive pill in the 1950s triggered huge social changes.
- Too little research was done on the psychological and emotional impact of the pill.
- Hormones were found to have direct effects on brain chemicals

– the neurotransmitters that control moods. This explains how hormones can make us feel sexy and loving or weepy and out of control.

- The hormonal impact on our brains is still largely ignored by doctors, leading to poor treatment.
- There is a list of questions that doctors need to ask to distinguish between the depressive symptoms caused by hormones and those that are the result of other causes.
- The most effective treatment for hormonal problems is the use of bio-identical hormones, which are not the same as those in HRT.

CHAPTER TWO

DEMYSTIFYING HORMONES

● ● ● ●

In the previous chapter we saw just how important it is for the medical profession to engage seriously with bio-identical hormones because the artificial versions they rely on can have the opposite effect to the natural ones. To date, the medical profession has been very conservative and reticent to change their prescribing habits, even though BHRT has been around for a long time. Fortunately, in 2018 in the UK, NICE (National Institute for Health and Care Excellence) guidelines for menopausal symptoms changed. NICE now recommends micronised progesterone and oestradiol (both body-identical hormones) for the menopause.

To take charge of your hormonal health, you need to begin by becoming familiar with your hormonal rhythms. I cannot reiterate enough how important this is. It continues to surprise me when I encounter women in my practice who have little knowledge of their own bodies. It's got nothing to do with education; I have seen CEOs and politicians, journalists and housewives. You can have stacks of academic qualifications and yet still find the workings of your body as mysterious and complex as a quantum computer.

We seem to either take our biology for granted when all is working well, or feel doomed and at the mercy of our moods, cycles and ill health when hormonal balance and harmony have been lost. There is certainly a hunger for knowledge, as the many books and other materials on hormones testify, but theoretical knowledge is not enough. My message to the patients in my practice has always been to be empowered and take control.

Be your own research subject. Keep a record of changes in your mood and emotions and see what kind of a pattern shows up. This was how Dr Katharina Dalton (mentioned briefly in the introduction) identified a link between PMS, mental health and even criminal violence. She made the connection sixty years ago, yet it is still uncommon for doctors to think of hormones as a possible underlying factor in serious psychological problems.

How diaries can pinpoint emotional crisis and hormone link

Poet and novelist Sylvia Plath kept a diary from the age of eight that later described her attempts at suicide, her electric shock treatment, her psychoanalysis and her tumultuous and even violent relationship with the poet Ted Hughes. Her novel *The Bell Jar* describes her hyper focus on how to kill herself. She tried it with pills and finally succeeded by gassing herself in 1963 when she was just thirty. When she was eighteen, she wrote, with what turned out to be remarkable prescience: 'If I didn't have sex organs, I wouldn't waver on the brink of nervous emotion and tears all the time.'

In 1990, an article by Catherine Thompson in the literary magazine *Triquarterly*, titled 'Dawn Poems in Blood: Sylvia Plath and PMS', made similar connections between Sylvia's intense emotional states and times of changing hormones. It seems as if Sylvia could have been suffering from premenstrual dysphoric disorder (PMDD), a severe form of PMS caused by wildly fluctuating hormones, specifically low progesterone and possibly oestrogen peaks, which brings in its wake a profoundly negative emotional state.

Sylvia had recorded in her diary symptoms we now recognise as cyclical PMS: unexplained tears, impulsiveness, inappropriate angry outbursts, hypersensitivity to offence, intense appetite changes. She was chronically plagued with cramps, insomnia, low mood, headaches, itchy skin, tinnitus, conjunctivitis, heart palpitations and sinus infections.

These symptoms can, through her diary, be tied to her hormonal cycle, with her most extreme emotional outbursts taking place in the luteal phase (the week before her period), when both progesterone and oestrogen could be low. That was when she fell out with close friends and relatives, ruined family holidays with emotional outbursts and destroyed Ted's treasured Shakespeare collection.

Her pregnancies exaggerated both her behaviour and her emotions. She breastfed both her babies for at least six months, and, from her journals, seems to have been particularly vulnerable to powerful depressive periods shortly after she weaned them, when hormone levels would have dropped sharply. In June 1962, she drove her car off the road, apparently in a compulsion to end her life.

The work Catherine Thompson has done in documenting and linking Sylvia's journals and poetry to her hormonal cycle gives us an extraordinary example of the interweaving of one woman's mind, mood and hormones.

There is a peculiar twist at the end of this tragic tale. A week before her death, Sylvia wrote to her mother telling her she was due to see a female doctor. That was most likely Dr Dalton. We can't know if she would have benefited from progesterone therapy, but we do know that, like many other women who have suffered from severe PMS, she found relief from her depression in pregnancy, when she was flush with progesterone, and that afterwards, when her hormones plummeted, she suffered from postnatal depression. Progesterone and individualised hormone balancing could certainly have taken the edge off her symptoms. If Sylvia had managed to visit Dr Dalton, I suspect that she would have given her an explanation, bringing hope and understanding, along with progesterone therapy.

It's very clear that the work of Dr Dalton and Thompson discovered a valuable way of connecting the dots and pointing to the real cause of our negative emotions and mood swings. But tragically it has had very little impact on treatment. The result is that hormones are still poorly understood by the GPs responsible for our health. Dalton was a medical expert and pioneer in hormone therapy, yet today she has few followers. Symptoms of hormonal issues are often cyclical or occur at times when women are hormonally challenged, such as post-partum (after birth) or during the perimenopause. How can such an obvious clue about what may be going on still be largely ignored?

That's why keeping track of your own cycles and noting the impact they have on how you feel and behave is a logical way of discovering what treatment you might benefit from. That makes this a good place to tell you a bit more about the hormone family. Oestrogen, progesterone and testosterone are obviously key members, but there are others that can play an important role for some people. So which are the hormones we women – and yes, also men – are driven by?

Meet the family

Oestrogen: the powerful female hormones

Oestrogen is the name for a group of hormones. Women produce three different types of oestrogen throughout their lifetime: oestradiol, oestrone and oestriol. These define us from birth to death and contribute to our female development and sexual characteristics, turning us into the women we become. Oestradiol is the principal oestrogen for women and is linked to emotional and physical well-being throughout our lives. It is closely associated with the feel-good brain chemicals such as serotonin and dopamine.

Oestrogen is essential for optimal brain function and helps us sleep, feel calm and be happy. It can be a blessing or a bane as it naturally ebbs and flows through the various phases of our lives. Oestrogen can make us feel and look great, think and focus well, and help us sleep and relax. But if it is too dominant or becomes out of balance with the other hormones, it may be disruptive and cause us anxiety. The amounts in our bodies diminish after menopause, but it never abandons us completely.

Progesterone: the calming pregnancy hormone

Progesterone is another feel-good hormone. It is the brain's sedative or tranquilliser, an anti-anxiety and mellowing agent. Its calming effect can reverse the effects of oestrogen dominance. Equilibrium between progesterone and oestrogen is the key to well-being. Both hormones affect our menstrual cycle, fertility, mood and metabolism. They act as a pair and belong together. Where oestrogen goes, progesterone must follow. Bio-identical progesterone can be mood-enhancing and works as a natural antidepressant. It increases the calming neurotransmitter GABA (gamma-aminobutyric acid), bringing relief to symptoms caused by hormonal imbalances.

Testosterone: the confident hormone

This hormone is falsely understood to be the supreme male hormone. Wrong! It is also a female hormone, and women produce it in their ovaries and adrenal glands. The only difference is that men have about ten to a hundred times more testosterone than women. Every woman needs testosterone, which can arouse sexual desire and increase libido. It also helps with assertiveness, confidence and physical strength. Testosterone makes bones and muscles strong. Too much testosterone in women can cause bad temper and aggression. It can also bring on acne and excessive body hair, while too little can cause loss of confidence and fatigue.

DHEA (dehydroepiandrosterone): the feel-good hormone

Produced in the brain and adrenal glands, this life-affirming hormone gives drive, enthusiasm and a zest for life. DHEA may ultimately turn into testosterone and oestrogen via the 'steroid pathway' (see pp.33–5), a clever way for the body to replace a hormone that has become depleted. DHEA is the most abundant hormone in youth and wanes to nothing in old age. It makes sense to want to preserve this hormone and its energising effect for as long as possible.

Thyroid: the metabolism and energy hormones

The thyroid gland at the base of the neck produces a pair of hormones, T4 (thyroxine) and T3 (liothyronine), which work together to influence practically every cell in the body. T4 is inert and needs to be turned into T3 to have an effect. The pair help to maintain your sanity, energy and metabolism. If you don't feel like your normal self and are succumbing to depression, lethargy and weight gain, it is quite possible that you are suffering from too little of these hormones, which can be easily remedied by a supplement of T4. It is worth knowing, though, that some people don't benefit from a T4 supplement because a genetic glitch means they are unable to convert it to T3.

Pregnenolone: the memory hormone

Pregnenolone enhances a healthy cognitive function and helps you to remember the names of your friends! It is also nicknamed 'the mother hormone' as it converts to progesterone in the body, which can then make most of the other 'steroid' hormones.

Oxytocin: the love hormone

This is the bonding, cuddling, nurturing hormone. It is also closely associated with dopamine and serotonin, which are feel-good neurotransmitters that work in the brain. Oxytocin is the hormone that increases uterine contraction during pregnancy and stimulates lactation. It is the primary bonding hormone between mother and baby, and between father and baby.

Where do hormones come from?

So, if you want your emotional issues to be taken seriously, it helps to know about the steroid pathway, which is where the main steroid hormones come from. All hormones are made from cholesterol. This may come as a surprise to you, as cholesterol is more commonly linked with heart disease. It's used to make pregnenolone – mostly in the adrenal glands, which are just above the kidneys in your lower back. This hormone provides the raw material for progesterone, which is the starting point for all the others; just follow the arrows in the diagram opposite and you can see.

Progesterone then makes testosterone, as well as the stress hormone cortisol. It may also come as a surprise to learn that testosterone is what the body uses to make the classically female hormone oestrogen. Your body sometimes makes use of this interchangeability to restore a balance or deal with a crisis. So if you are very stressed, your body will turn progesterone into the stress-reducing hormone cortisol. When men hit middle age, their testosterone can be used to make oestrogen. One effect of this is to create more belly fat.

All steroid hormones are produced in our adrenals, ovaries or testes. If you look at the diagram, you can see that all the steroid hormones evolve from cholesterol via pregnenolone. Pregnenolone is not a true hormone but is the starting material for all of the steroid hormones. Through biosynthesis, it becomes one of the five different types of steroid hormones (represented by different shades in the diagram): glucorticoids such as cortisol; mineralcorticoids such as aldosterone; androgens such as testosterone; oestrogens such as oestradiol; and progestogens such as progesterone. These are just some of the hormones we produce naturally, and which contribute to our mental and physical well-being. As there are continuous surges of hormones throughout our lifetime, we may experience hormonal deficiencies or imbalances, which may cause us significant distress. Should this occur, a doctor can prescribe bio-identical hormones to rebalance or replace our hormones.

THE STEROID PATHWAY

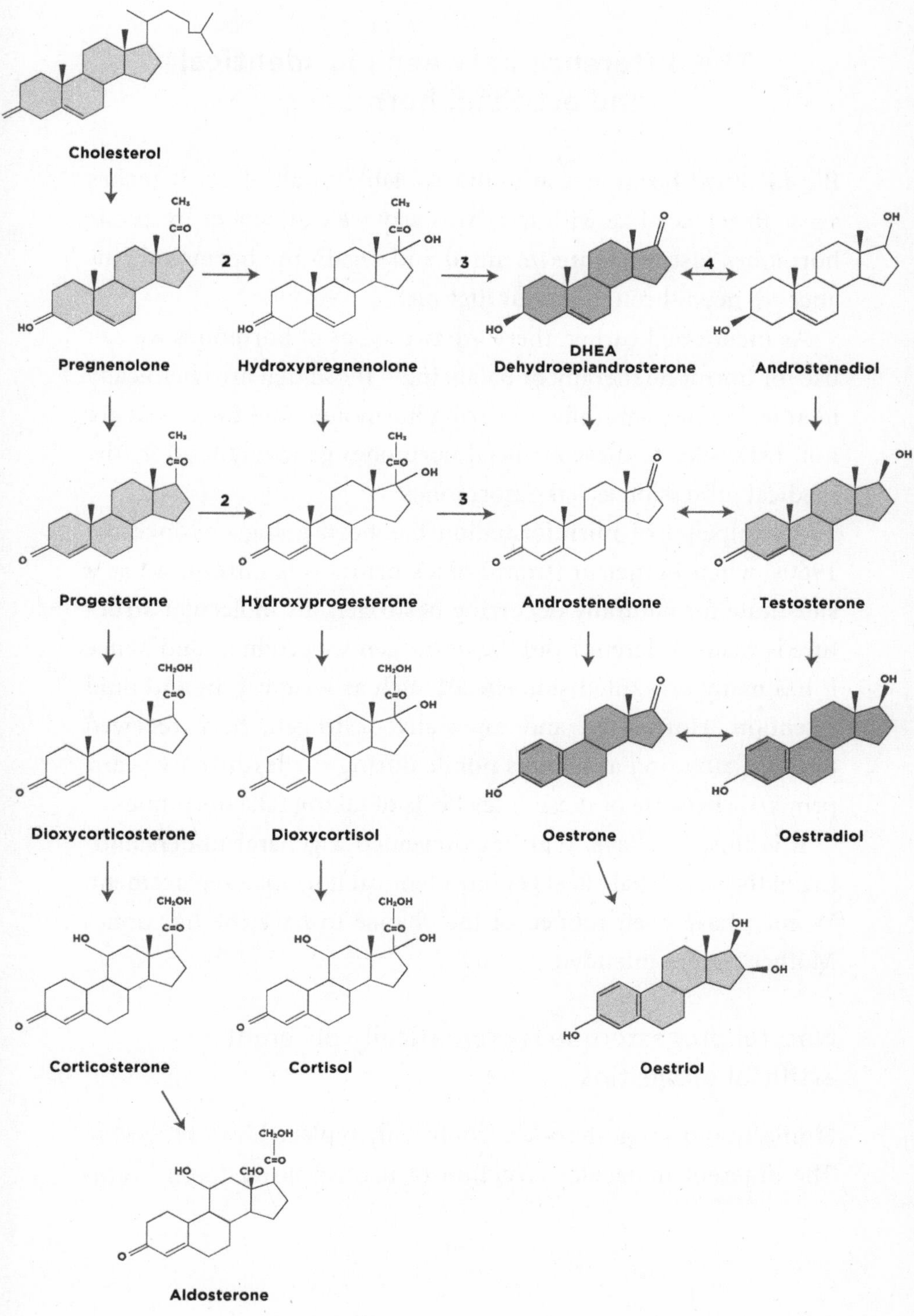

Cholesterol

Pregnenolone → 2 → **Hydroxypregnenolone** → 3 → **DHEA Dehydroepiandrosterone** ← 4 → **Androstenediol**

Progesterone → 2 → **Hydroxyprogesterone** → 3 → **Androstenedione** ↔ **Testosterone**

Dioxycorticosterone   **Dioxycortisol**   **Oestrone** ↔ **Oestradiol**

Corticosterone   **Cortisol**   **Oestriol**

Aldosterone

The difference between bio-identical and artificial hormones

Bio-identical hormones are now available to all of us. It makes sense to replace like with like. This way we can benefit from our hormones just as nature intended and regain the hormonal balance we need throughout our lifetime.

As mentioned earlier, there are two types of hormones we can use for hormone therapy or balancing – those that are chemically identical to our naturally occurring hormones, and those that are not. Let's refer to these artificial hormones generally used by the medical profession as 'fake' hormones.

A campaign of misinformation has been going on since the 1960s, when Premarin (from horse's urine) was introduced as a substitute for naturally occurring oestrogen. Its molecular structure is vastly different from the oestrogen we produce, and hence it has many unwanted side effects, such as weight gain and fluid retention. Hormones, and especially oestrogen, have received negative attention at various points during the last twenty years, primarily because of these side effects of taking fake hormones.

It is this, I believe, that has prevented a general understanding of the beneficial effects of bio-identical hormone replacement. Women have been robbed of the chance to have the hormones Mother Nature intended.

Natural progesterone is dramatically different to artificial progestins

Similarly, our progesterone is commonly replaced by a progestin. The different molecular structure of natural progesterone compared with progestin means that they will have significantly different effects on any recipient.

We have known for over fifty years that hormones play a major role in our moods and emotions. However, until recently we didn't believe that they had a direct effect on the brain, due to the blood–brain barrier, which protects the brain from bacteria and toxins swimming in our bloodstream. But in the last twenty years it has become clear that hormones not only do directly affect the brain, they are also produced inside the brain, where they are known as 'neurosteroids'.

You just have to look at the diagram of a molecule of natural progesterone (below) to see that there is a significant difference between its structure and that of the synthetic version beside it, known as progestin. This fake hormone – also known as Provera, or MPA (medroxyprogesterone acetate) – stops the conversion of natural progesterone to another hormone, allopregnanolone, which protects brain cells and is a natural tranquilliser with anti-stress effects. Progestin is the conventional substitute for progesterone, used in regular HRT and the contraceptive pill. Confusingly, it is frequently referred to in scientific studies as progesterone. This inaccuracy matters, because in the world of hormones, very small differences can produce big effects.

BIO-IDENTICAL
Progesterone

SYNTHETIC
Progestin
(Medroxypregesteroneacetate)

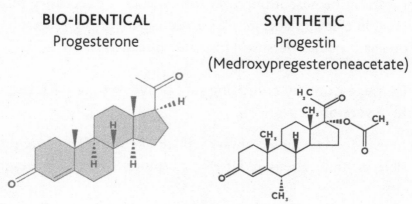

It is clear from the other pair shown below that a small difference can have a big effect. The diagram shows bio-identical oestrogen and bio-identical testosterone, which differ by just a single hydrogen atom. Yet oestrogen is responsible for defining female features such as breasts, while testosterone is what makes men more muscled and masculine.

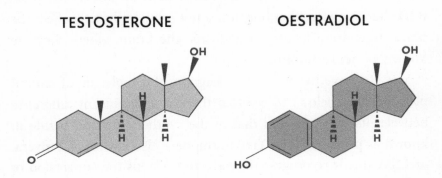

So, when the molecules in natural oestrogen and testosterone are more alike than those in natural and artificial progesterone molecules, you shouldn't be surprised that progesterone and progestin can have very different effects. In fact, they often have the opposite effect. For instance, progesterone is the hormone produced in large amounts in pregnancy and is given to women having IVF treatment because it improves their chances of becoming pregnant. In contrast, doctors are warned against giving progestin to pregnant women because it can cause miscarriage!

Damage done by confusing real progesterone with the fake version

In my view, we should always replace like with like where possible; anything else is an inferior substitute. Synthetic progestins are used almost everywhere as a replacement for progesterone, but they can have very negative effects on our physical and mental health.

An example of the harm this did can be seen in the way a senior executive in women's health research and associate professor at Yale University, Florence Haseltine, handled her own menopause. In 1990, at the age of forty-eight, she arranged to have her womb and ovaries removed.

She had been plagued by hot flushes and would have taken oestrogen to treat them but knew that she would have to combine it with 'a progesterone' to reduce the risk of developing cancer of the womb, which she was not prepared to do. In actual fact, the negative reaction she described refers to progestin and not progesterone. I am well aware of the unpleasant side effects of progestin, especially on mood, but I have very seldom encountered a strong negative reaction to progesterone. On the contrary, progesterone is the happy and calming hormone that can be a life-changer for many women.

Sadly, even today women are advised to have a total hysterectomy (uterus and ovaries surgically removed) so that they can take oestrogen replacement therapy alone. There are so many unnecessary hysterectomies done without considering using progesterone replacement therapy first, or the psychological consequences for a woman when she has her uterus and ovaries removed.

HRT is given in a number of different ways. The one that shows the effect of progestin most clearly contains just oestrogen for the first two weeks of a cycle, followed by oestrogen and progestin for the second two. Those second two weeks, which would normally be a time of calmness, are often described as being deeply unpleasant. It was this feeling that Professor Haseltine was prepared to lose her womb to avoid.

This confusion among medical professionals continues to this day. In Chapter Five, I discuss the excessive use of hysterectomies because of the damaging lack of awareness of the value of maintaining an intact womb, and the need for proper hormonal support after it has been removed.

Scientific backing for bio-identical benefits

As you might expect, there is now a lot of evidence that progestins can cause a range of other problems, including heart disease and cancer, yet in the UK alone the number of prescriptions for progestins is over a million, while just 50,000 are written for progesterone.

This is due to the remarkable refusal of the obstetrics and gynaecological community to recognise the difference and its implications. So, I am very encouraged to learn that a growing number of women don't believe these experts. A few years ago, a study presented at the Endocrine Society's 97th annual meeting found that, despite warnings that there was not enough scientific proof – i.e. double-blind placebo studies – regarding the efficacy and safety of BHRT, use of bio-identical hormones was steadily increasing. Almost half of the prescriptions for menopausal hormone therapy in the USA are now 'custom compounded bio-identical hormones.[1]

I am delighted by women's good sense and am confident that there is convincing evidence for the safety and effectiveness of bio-identical hormones.

---

1   The Endocrine Society, 'Pharmacist survey shows huge growth in compounded menopausal hormone therapy', 6 March 2015. Available at: https://www.eurekalert.org/pub_releases/2015-03/tes-pss030515.php.

If you are setting out to become acquainted with your hormones, it is worth knowing about the favourable research to counter the knee-jerk negative reactions you may encounter. In fact, when studies are done, they usually show bio-identical hormones as safer than fake hormones.

Nearly twenty years ago, a very big study on the side effects of HRT, discussed later, found that the combination of artificial progesterone (progestin) and artificial oestrogen (derived from horses' urine) had links to cancer and heart disease. Shockingly, this combo is still being prescribed today. Even so, it is bio-identical hormones that are routinely dismissed with comments such as this, made in a medical journal relatively recently: 'The use of bio-identical hormones is based on misconceptions and unfounded claims that they are more natural and safer than approved hormone therapy.'[2]

Previously I wrote about the growing evidence that bio-identical progesterone is beneficial for the brain and artificial progestins are not. Even so, the Endocrine Society felt able to assert in 2016 that 'evidence demonstrating a benefit of micronized progesterone (the most widely available bio-identical form) on clinical outcomes is lacking'.[3] The politest response I can manage is that the society doesn't know what it is talking about.

---

2   L. Pattimakiel and H. L. Thacker, 'Bioidentical hormone therapy: clarifying the misconceptions', *Cleveland Clinic Journal of Medicine*, December 2011, 78(12):829–36.

3   www.endo-society.org/advocacy/policy/upload/BH_position_Statement_final_10_25_06_w_Header.pdf

Journal *Nature* finds artificial progestins raise risk of breast cancer

The idea that progesterone is safer and more effective in relation to cancer than progestins received strong support from a paper in top science journal *Nature* in 2015. It reported what scientists had found when they used high-powered microscopes to see what bio-identical oestrogen and progesterone actually did inside a cancer cell.[4] This is where hormonal effects take place.

The researchers found that the specialised molecule (receptor) that naturally responds to progesterone was actively knocking out breast cancer cells. The result, in the cautious language of a science journal, was that a 'unique gene expression programme' was activated 'that is associated with good clinical outcome'.

Not only did *Nature* provide a plausible reason why progesterone could be protecting against breast cancer, the report also commented: 'There is compelling evidence that inclusion of a progestin – especially Provera [the one used for years in HRT] increases the risk of breast cancer.'

Shockingly, patients have been misled about oestrogen in very much the same way. As a result, many women have become afraid of it. This would seem a bizarre belief about something that is essential for life, inherently female and vital for our brain function and mental well-being. But it is perfectly understandable in light of the misinformation women have been getting.

The readiness of the medical profession to expose women, especially those with psychological and emotional problems, to

---

4   H. Mohammed et al., 'Progesterone receptor modulates ERα action in breast cancer', *Nature*, July 2015, 16, 523(7560):313–17.

damaging aggressive treatment with these inherently problematic 'conventional' or 'synthetic' hormones has a long and disreputable history.

How claims about the benefits of HRT kept changing

The information patients and doctors have been given about the fake hormones has been remarkably inconsistent and confusing. To begin with they were presented as a remarkable, life-changing breakthrough, but then stories started to emerge about the dangerous side effects. Always, however, there is a new, improved version on the horizon. At the beginning of the 1960s, the contraceptive pill was the wonderful new breakthrough and women were demanding that the artificial hormones it contained be available to them. A decade later, in the 1970s, the demand was for HRT, which also contained synthetic hormones.

Our enthusiasm was understandable. We didn't want to be controlled by our hormones. We wanted to be free to continue to work, to embrace our professions and decide when we would become pregnant. We wanted to maintain our energy, libido and vitality into our postmenopausal years. We wanted to be liberated from what society demanded of 'a conventional woman' and from the tyranny of our hormones. But the hormone story could have been so different if only largely commercial organisations hadn't poured money into researching and promoting the more dangerous artificial versions. We could have benefited from safer and more effective bio-identical hormones from the beginning.

The synthetic hormone revolution really took off with the arrival of the oral contraceptive pill in 1960. Women felt they had found their route to sexual liberation and a new-found freedom. Doctors, the media, the women's rights movement, everyone was on board with this empowering new treatment. What went wrong? The answer lies in the history of how hormones first became available.

In the early part of the twentieth century, a remarkable group of ingenious chemists working in the States were investigating ways to scale up production of the steroid hormones (oestrogen, progesterone and cortisol), which had only recently been isolated from animal sources – testes, ovaries, placentas and so on. To make them on an industrial scale, a cheap and readily available source was needed, and the hunt was on for a plant source.

They were looking at a type of plant known to contain phytosterols. These plants have a similar chemical structure to cholesterol, which is the starting point for producing sex hormones in the body. Plants in the family include soy, some lilies, yucca and yams.

One of the chemists, a man named Russell Marker, identified a giant Mexican yam root as a possible source raw material. He smuggled 50 lb of it back to the USA for further research and successfully produced a bio-identical form of progesterone from it.[5] This was the first time a bio-identical hormone had been recreated, replicating a human hormone. Unfortunately, beneficial as it could have been for patients, there was a serious drawback. Being a natural product, it couldn't be patented and so was not going to make the kind of money the drug companies expected. The same was true for the other bio-identical versions of hormones the yam could be used to produce. (For more information on the history of

---

5 Mandy Redig, 'Yams of Fortune: the (Uncontrolled) Birth of Oral Contraceptives', *Journal of Young Investigators*, Issue 7, February 2003. Available at: http://legacy.jyi.org/volumes/volume6/issue7/features/redig.html.

progesterone, see the Recommended Reading section at the end of the book.)

However, Marker's discovery kick-started the pharmaceutical companies into developing versions that were slightly different from the natural ones and so could be patented. This work culminated in the pharmaceutical holy grail of an oral contraceptive containing hormone compounds that were similar to progesterone and oestrogen, but with a slightly different structure. The bio-identical versions were pushed into obscurity.

How the menopause became medicalised

In 1966, American gynaecologist Robert Wilson wrote *Feminine Forever*, which became a number-one bestseller. He assured women they could remain eternally young and sexually attractive if they replaced their diminishing natural hormones with artificial oestrogen. They need no longer succumb to the 'living decay' of ageing.

His promise of this elixir of youth brought hope to many women, but the hormone therapy he recommended set the tone for what was to come. Premarin, the synthetic substitute for oestrogen, was going to free us from deregulated hormones. But it turned out to be another example in an unfortunate history of women being manipulated and exploited. Society had turned a natural stage of life – the menopause – into a disease.

When we have a disease, we look for drugs to treat it. Seeing the menopause as a disease was the beginning of its medicalisation and the continuation of the exploitation of women's health issues. Of course, it makes sense to replenish our diminishing hormones to maintain our health and quality of life, but doing this using inferior synthetic substitutes eventually led to a fear of oestrogen and distrust of our own natural hormones. It wasn't long before women suffered the unpleasant side effects of synthetic oestrogen; not only headaches, but weight gain, bloating and mood swings became a common problem, and an increase in female cancers was on the rise. Why?

The promise of *Feminine Forever* was never delivered because, as well as being a poor mimic of natural oestrogen, the Premarin that Robert Wilson and his fellow proponents of HRT recommended was taken on its own, without the support of progesterone in any form. This 'unopposed' synthetic oestrogen resulted in a large increase in endometrial and uterine cancers. This should not have been surprising, as oestrogen is a growth stimulant, making the lining of the womb thicken, a change that can become cancerous.

What Wilson failed to mention in his book was that he had a considerable financial interest in the promotion of unopposed oestrogen. He had founded an organisation that was funded by the drug companies that made Premarin: 'His book was sold as expert advice but really it was one large advertisement.'[6]

Subsequent research proposed that 'progesterone' (as progestins were often wrongly described) be added to 'oppose' the unwanted side effects of oestrogen on the uterus. Throughout the 1980s and 90s, the combined synthetic Premarin/Provera HRT became the recommended treatment for menopause, despite all the risks now increasingly being recognised.

Encouraged by the pharmaceutical companies, the focus of the medical profession shifted from the promise of eternal youth

6   Randi Hutter-Epstein, *Aroused: The history of hormones and how they control just about everything,* W. W. Norton & Company, 2018

to prevention, with the companies' PR departments promoting this synthetic HRT as a way to stave off heart disease, stroke and osteoporosis. Doctors should prescribe 'hormones for all women for the rest of their lives', a slogan propagated by the pharmaceutical industry to convince women that it was the right thing to do.

Back then, this preventative medicine was considered the 'gold standard' of good treatment, with its promise of maintaining women in the best possible health, but today it has become the scourge of women's health. This was the beginning of the distrust and fear of hormones, specifically oestrogen. Doctors and patients alike equated natural hormones with the 'fake' synthetic ones that were invariably prescribed.

Oestrogen becomes dangerous

At the time, not everyone accepted that this approach to hormone therapy was a good idea. Controversy and mistrust remained as HRT went mainstream. Women were hearing conflicting information about positive and negative impacts. Anecdotally, patients and doctors suspected HRT to be behind the rise of female-related cancers.

After much lobbying from the women's movement, in 1993 the American government funded an extensive study called the Women's Health Initiative (WHI), involving 161,808 women between the ages of fifty and seventy-nine. This was supposed to last decades and provide definitive answers but was halted prematurely in 2002 due to ethical concerns. The results that were coming in were alarming: a dramatic increase in breast cancer, as well as strokes and heart attacks, amongst the women taking the HRT combination of Premarin and Provera.

As Premarin was then the top-selling drug in the USA, this was a potential disaster for the pharmaceutical company that produced it. However, women were no longer being fooled. What had long been anticipated and feared was finally proven: synthetic hormones were deleterious to a woman's health. This was a disastrous result for women, even more so as the medical community was not in favour of natural hormones and women were left in the lurch, with nowhere to turn to find out about the existing safer options for HRT.

The results of the WHI study have been contentious ever since, causing chaos and disarray among doctors over hormone treatment protocols, and disappointment and disillusionment amongst women. The study created a climate of fear surrounding hormones and HRT. This anxiety spread to all other forms of hormone balancing or replacement therapy. Once cancer became falsely associated with hormones, it was hugely difficult to educate women about the value of their own hormones, and the fact that natural hormones actually protect us from stroke, heart disease and cancer. Sadly, the medical profession made no attempt to recognise or acknowledge the difference between naturally occurring hormones and synthetic ones, so the benefits of using bio-identical oestrogen and progesterone to treat hormonal imbalances, improve mental well-being and reduce the incidence of cancer and heart disease were lost to mainstream medicine.

The oral contraceptive pill: is it safe?

The revelations about HRT raised questions about the safety of the oral contraceptive pill, which contained synthetic hormones no different to those in HRT. For the last fifty years, doctors have routinely prescribed the OCP to girls as young as twelve. It is prescribed not only to prevent pregnancy, but to treat irregular periods, mood swings and acne, and to halt unwanted periods either temporarily or for years at a time. It has even been given for PMS symptoms. Research now shows that like HRT, it may increase the symptoms it is trying to relieve.

Mood swings and depression are very common side effects of the OCP. Because of these side effects, it is impossible to say that the pill is safe for all young girls and women needing contraception. In fact, for many it doesn't look like a healthy option at all to be taking synthetic hormones.

Does the OCP affect mental health?

It really is time we understood the role hormones play in disturbing or improving our moods and emotions. Recent research suggests that the use of artificial hormones in contraceptive pills could be contributing to reports of increasing levels of depression and anxiety.

The OCP is often prescribed to improve mood swings. Yet it has been linked with depression, resulting in an increased reliance on antidepressants. A recent review described a link between the contraceptive pill and depression, and other examples of how the beneficial effects of natural progesterone in the brain can be blocked by the fake progestins.[7] Therefore, if we master our natural hormones, we should be better able to control our moods and emotions without the fear of unwanted side effects.

In 2016, the American Medical Association published a study of over one million Danish women that found an association

---

7   *JAMA Psychiatry,* 2016; 73(11):1154-1162. doi:10.1001/jamapsychiatry.2016.2387

between use of the contraceptive pill, diagnosis of depression and subsequent antidepressant use.[8]

Another Danish study of over a thousand women aged between fifteen and nineteen found an association between going on the pill and becoming depressed and attempting suicide. None of the subjects was depressed at the start of the study, but the younger they were when a negative mood set in, the greater their risk of suicide. Adolescent girls seemed more vulnerable to this risk. According to the study: 'Use of hormonal contraception, especially among adolescents, was associated with subsequent use of antidepressants and a first diagnosis of depression, suggesting depression as a potential adverse effect of hormonal contraceptive use.'[9]

The study found that when compared with girls not on the pill, those taking the OCP were more likely to be diagnosed with depression and to be prescribed an antidepressant. This risk was even greater for those given the progestin-only or 'mini' pill.

Bio-identical oestrogen and progesterone have a positive and protective effect on the brain. Oestrogen enhances mood by increasing serotonin, and progesterone promotes sleep and relaxation. Progesterone and its metabolite allopregnanolone are neuroprotective, as they help to adapt to stress or brain cell injury. Research has found that synthetic progestins can stop the normal hormonal ebb and flow and reduce the amount of natural hormones available – both changes that are likely to result in feelings of depression and anxiety.

8   Charlotte Wessel Skovlund et al., 'Association of Hormonal Contraception with Depression', *JAMA Psychiatry,* 2016, 73(11):1154–62. Available at: doi:10.1001/jamapsychiatry.2016.2387.

9   *JAMA Psychiatry,* 2016; 73(11):1154-1162. doi: 10.1001/jamapsychiatry.2016.2387

Can hormone treatment be the answer for mood swings?

The efficacy of using hormones to treat mood swings and depression has been known about for over seventy years, so why has it been ignored and the medical profession been encouraged instead to rely on drugs?

Panic followed the WHI findings and caused a sharp decline in HRT prescriptions during the first decade of the twenty-first century, with women once again suffering the consequences of hormonal imbalance. This has been closely mirrored by a dramatic increase in prescriptions of antidepressants to treat the symptoms of hormonal withdrawal such as mood swings and depression. This is not a coincidence. Sadly, the medical profession turned to antidepressants to combat the symptoms of menopause instead of searching for healthy and safer alternatives to treat hormonal imbalances.

Because there has been no distinction made between natural bio-identical hormones and synthetic HRT, women have been deprived of confidence in hormone therapy in general. In response to fears raised by the WHI findings, doctors, menopause societies and women's health experts now reach for antidepressants as the treatment of choice for hormone-related mood swings that can trigger PMS and postnatal depression. No drug is without side effects, and giving antidepressants as a treatment for symptoms that are due to a hormone deficiency or imbalance does women a great disservice.

This reliance on antidepressants is also causing the cash-strapped NHS to spend unnecessary millions. The shocking revelation that the number of antidepressant prescriptions has more than doubled in the last decade means that more than 67 million prescriptions are being issued every year, at a cost of £280 million per year and rising. Many of these prescriptions were undoubtedly unnecessary. The medical profession is letting us down, and we are letting our children down by not being better informed and not challenging the rationale for current medical wisdom.

When we ask the right questions and find the right answers, we will be more likely to find the optimal hormone balance for healthy mind and body. At the same time, we need to consider our lifestyle, what role stress plays in our life, whether we are eating the right foods and living as well as possible in our environment.

So when we feel out of sorts or are moody or behaving irrationally, it would be good to ask ourselves, 'Why is this happening to me now? What's going on in my life to make me feel this way and how can I help myself to feel better?' Part of the answer may well involve hormones, and keeping a diary, as mentioned earlier, could help to identify the problem more precisely. But in order to do that properly, it helps if you have a sense of the way hormones change and fluctuate at various times through the life cycle. That's the topic of the next chapter.

SUMMARY OF KEY POINTS

- Get to know your normal hormonal rhythms by keeping a diary. Note how and when your emotions regularly change.
- Sylvia Plath's diaries pinpointed a link between her emotional crises and her unbalanced hormones.

- Progestins can cause a great deal of harm, yet are widely used by the medical profession. There is evidence that bio-identical hormones are much safer than synthetic hormones, yet as there is no clear differentiation made between fake and bio-identical hormones, all hormones have been tarred with the same brush.
- The first hormone to be made from a cheap and widely available source was natural progesterone. As this was naturally occurring, it could not be patented and therefore could not turn a profit. The profitable artificial version was made shortly afterwards.
- There is a huge difference between real and fake hormones; even if that difference seems tiny, the effects can be drastic.
- There are scientific studies supporting the use of bio-identical hormones.
- Artificial progestins raise the risk of breast cancer.
- The claims about HRT benefits kept changing as risks emerged, causing confusion for patients and medical professionals alike.
- The pill: promise of a brave new world.
- The menopause has become a medical problem to be treated with fake hormones.
- Oestrogen is linked to a cancer scare.
- The oral contraceptive pill is linked to a rise in depression in young women. Prescriptions for antidepressants have doubled.
- The failure to distinguish between real and fake hormones has been a disaster for women.

CHAPTER THREE

HORMONE RHYTHMS FROM BIRTH TO MATURITY

● ● ● ●

As we saw in the previous chapter, women's greater sensitivity to their hormonal rhythms has all too often been the excuse for treatments that promise much but turn out to be dangerous or the source of myths about hysteria and unreliability. In fact, our rhythms should be cause for celebration, a source of pride and wonder. The natural world is woven together with rhythms and cycles, from the tiny rhythms of breathing and heartbeats to the majestic progression of the earth around the sun, which itself is marked by the ebb and flow of the tides, the phases of the moon and the cycle of the seasons. Our hormones net us into all this.

The way technology shapes our lives now, however, means that we are mostly oblivious of this ever-changing natural parade that so dominated the lives of our ancestors. It is a detachment that has contributed on the macro scale to our growing environmental crisis, but there is a penalty for largely ignoring our bodies' micro circadian (daily) rhythms as well.

Familiar hormones such as insulin and testosterone are higher in the morning and decline towards evening, when melatonin starts to rise and promote sleep. But many more physical changes cycle through the day, such as heart rate, the strength of the immune and inflammatory responses and cell clean-up processes.

These largely unconscious processes are all part of our circadian rhythms that wax and wane on a 24-hour cycle and are run by a master controller in the brain known as SCN (nuclei or suprachiasmatic nucleus). This command centre also regulates the daily rhythms that we are more aware of such as sleeping and waking, feeling hungry or full, body temperature and the changing levels of our hormones.

But this is not a closed system, it can be disrupted by what is going on in the world around you. Things that disrupt your normal sleep/wake cycles, such as jet lag or working night shifts, can often result in weight gain. That's why shift workers face an increased risk for Type 2 diabetes, heart disease and cancer when appetite, digestion and metabolic processes are pushed out of sync with our 24-hour clock.[1]

But you don't have to be doing the night shift in a hospital or driving the night bus to be affected by rhythm shifts. Setting off early to work on the week days and then staying up late and sleeping in on weekends, then going to bed early to get back into the early waking rhythm in the week, sets you up for a mismatch between your circadian rhythm and your social sleep schedule And like more routine shift working, it cause similar metabolic changes.

The various elements of this rhythmic metabolic system make up a biological tangle of interconnecting pathways and feedback mechanisms, like the ecological webs that underpin forests,

---

1   G. Asher and P. Sassone-Corsi, 'Time for food: the intimate interplay between nutrition, metabolism and the circadian clock,' *Cell*, 2015, 161(1), 84-92.

coral reefs or the Arctic ice. You can see this in the way they can all influence ones another. Disrupted eating times with night shifts leads to weight gain, but disruption of our hormones can have the same effect.

We've seen that fluctuating hormones can produce depression and mood swings, but they also result in weight gain and problems with sleep. Oestrogen dominance (when progesterone levels are low) plays a big role along with other hormones, such as cortisol, leptin and insulin. Balancing all of them can help lose weight.[2]

Supplementing with progesterone can be particularly beneficial by affecting key points on this circuit. It lowers insulin which, when pushed up by the excess oestrogen, encourages weight gain. It also tunes up the thyroid gland, which in turn improves sleep, which then allows us to process food more effectively.

But such issues are rarely picked up in conventional diagnosis as changes in rhythms are not really on the medical radar, so it is not surprising that disruptions in the (mainly) female hormonal rhythms are also frequently ignored.

As an introduction to just how remarkable your hormonal system is, come on a tour that shows how it ebbs and flows through your brain, affecting its function and certain distinct parts during the different phases of our lives: from infancy through childhood to postmenopause. Hormones are ever present and elicit different feelings and reactions depending on what stage of life we are in and where we are in our hormone cycle.

From the earliest point of foetal brain development to the challenges of ageing, our human hormones are programmed to trigger and influence the way we engage with life. This is an intricate and complex process that we are only just beginning to understand,

---

2   https://gethealthyu.com/balance-4-hormones-want-lose-weight/

an understanding that will provide new answers to the question 'How can I help myself to master my health and well-being?'

Brain development and hormones

A female brain develops differently to a male brain in the womb. All this happens in the first eighteen weeks of pregnancy. In the beginning, all foetal brains look female, but triggered by both DNA and sex hormones, by the eighth week they begin to differ and develop into distinctly female or male.

Hormones flowing through the placenta from the mother enter the foetus's bloodstream. The female brain, under the influence of oestrogen, will develop more connections in the communication centres and areas where emotions are processed, such as the limbic area and prefrontal cortex (see p.60). Under the influence of testosterone, the male brain will develop a larger centre for sex and aggression at the cost of losing communication cells.

Are we surprised to learn that women's brains have bigger communication centres and men's brains have bigger centres for sex and aggression? Not really. That is why we are different. Although men and women have the same hormones, it is the total amount of hormones and how they work that make us female and male.

Neuroscience research suggests that male brains are 'structured to facilitate connections between perception and coordinated action', whereas the female brain 'facilitates communication between analytical and intuitive processing modes'.[3] I think some of us can relate to this anecdotally: it often seems that men are more rational and women more intuitive. I realise that these are stereotypes,

---

3   Louann Brizendine MD, *The Female Brain,* Transworld, 2009.

but there appears to be some neurodevelopmental truth behind them.

A woman's brain does not actually differ structurally from a man's. Both have the same number of neurons, but the female brain is smaller because the cells are more compact. However, as we have seen, some areas in the female brain may be larger, such as those involved with empathy and intuition. The areas that are larger in men include those handling sexual pursuit and for sensing danger.

Brain function and hormones

What role does the brain play in shaping our mood, emotions and personality?

Scientists have long known that our amazing brain is the master control centre for all our physical and biological activities, but it has only recently become clear that much of what it does is strongly affected by our sex hormones, and that it is the key to an optimally functioning endocrine (hormonal) system.

A recent review of brain scanning studies[4] showed that sex hormones were involved in processes in both the cortex – the part of the brain where thinking and planning goes on, located at the front just below the skull – and the area below that (subcortical), which is involved in processing emotions. These processes include the limbic system, where both fear and pleasure are processed, the hypothalamus, which controls food and sexual appetites, and the hippocampus, which is vital for memory. These regions have

---

4   S. Toffoletto et al., 'Emotional and cognitive functional imaging of estrogen and progesterone effects in the female human brain: a systematic review', *Psychoneuroendocrinology*, December 2014, 50:28–52.
Available at: https://www.ncbi.nlm.nih.gov/pubmed/25222701.

receptors all over them that respond to oestrogen and progesterone.

The prefrontal cortex is a part of the brain that contributes to personality development, planning and making decisions. Oestrogen is involved here in the way we respond to stress and how active the immune system is, as well as how sharp memory and attention are. Oestrogen is important for the executive functions of the prefrontal cortex, specifically cognition.[5] It is this midlife decline in cognition that concerns many women in the menopause transition. But research shows us just how complicated all this is, as everyone responds to hormones in their own unique way. For instance, while some women benefit from getting more oestrogen during menopause, some do better with less and some aren't affected either way.[6] This is another example of how different we all are and the importance of individualising each treatment regime. What is good for one person may be detrimental for another, even though symptoms may be the same.

However, it's clear that the prefrontal cortex helps us to be sociable and reasonable in our behaviour. It inhibits uncontrolled emotions and impulses and is bigger in women than in men.

Oestrogen fluctuations – the highs and lows of the hormone – may be the cause of oversensitive or irrational behaviour. There are times when we may cry or overreact to minor events, such as getting emotional or teary over a TV soap story. This is more likely to happen in women, but you may have noticed that men can be similarly affected.

---

5   See: http://www.thescienceofpsychotherapy.com/prefrontal-cortex/.

6   S. Shanmugan and C. Neill Epperson, 'Estrogen and the Prefrontal Cortex: Towards a New Understanding Estrogen's Effects on Executive Functions in the Menopause Transition', *Human Brain Mapping, March, 2014, 35(3):847–65. Available at: https://www.ncbi.nlm.nih.gov/pmc/articles/PMC4104582/.*

Becoming overemotional and easily shedding tears is not uncommon in men with low testosterone levels, because it makes them more responsive to oestrogen. It is also more common among older men, because testosterone levels decline with age and the smaller amount that remains may then be converted to oestrogen. Our emotions are all generated in the prefrontal cortex, which is highly sensitive to hormone fluctuations, in men as well as women.

Research also shows that the decline in oestrogen levels in post-menopausal women may be associated with lapses in short-term memory (controlled by the hypothalamus). I'm sure we have all experienced that feeling of walking into a room and forgetting what we were looking for, or forgetting names of friends or every-day objects and places. What we might not realise is that it is our diminishing hormones that could be the cause.

We are just scratching the surface in our understanding of the brain, and neuroendocrinology is now a booming area of research. It is being driven by increasingly sophisticated MRI scanners, which allow scientists to watch areas of the brain light up when certain emotions are aroused. The hope is that this research will improve our understanding of how emotions are created and controlled.

The limbic system is the brain's gratification system or emotional centre. It is made up of the amygdala, hippocampus, thalamus and hypothalamus. It deals with emotions, fear, memories and arousal. The highest concentration of neurotransmitters, such as serotonin and dopamine, are found in this part of the brain, together with many oestrogen receptors.[7] These neurotransmitters are the chemical messengers that send signals throughout the

---

7   G. J. ter Horst, 'Estrogen in the limbic system', *Vitamins and Hormones*, 2010, 82:319–38. Available at: https://www.ncbi.nlm.nih.gov/pubmed/20472146.

limbic system, assigning an emotional value to objects and situations and, under the influence of oestrogen, guiding our mood, emotions and behaviour.

LIMBIC SYSTEM

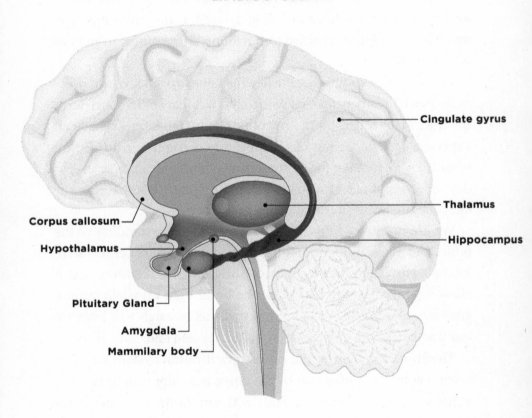

The amygdala is smaller in women than in men. It turns on the 'fight-or-flight' response by releasing stress-related hormones such as adrenaline and cortisol, which can make you anxious or fearful when you are feeling under threat. This is the area that attaches emotional significance to events and memories. It is where feelings of anger, fear and sadness are processed; it also controls aggression. The amygdala is studded with receptors that respond to oestrogen, progesterone and testosterone.

The hypothalamus, although small, approximately the size of an almond, has a major role in influencing the endocrine and nervous system[8] in both women and men. Most importantly, it is responsible for establishing equilibrium (what we doctors call homeostasis) in the body. To maintain this balance, the hypothalamus, together with an even smaller gland (about the size of a pea) called the pituitary, attached to it at the bottom, controls the production of many of the body's hormones and their actions.

The hormones that the hypothalamus and the pituitary gland activate include those from our thyroid and adrenal glands, and from the ovaries and testes. Oestrogen stimulates the nerve cells or neurons in the hypothalamus; it's the mediator or facilitator of action. A study from 2003 reports on the importance of oestrogen and its multiple effects on brain function, such as cognition, neuroprotection and the improvement of depression and other psychiatric disorders.[9] Given the important and widespread role that oestrogen plays in affecting brain function, it's not surprising that fluctuating levels can have a dramatic and sometimes unpleasant impact.

The brain's communication and translation network

There is an area at the base of the brain where most of our emotional responses are regulated, and it is here that the neurosteroids

---

8   M. J. Kelly et al., 'Estrogen signaling in the hypothalamus', *Vitamins and Hormones*, 2005, 71:123–45. Available at: https://www.ncbi.nlm.nih.gov/pubmed/16112267.

9   W. J. Cutter et al., 'Oestrogen, brain function, and neuropsychiatric disorders', *Journal of Neurology*, Neurosurgery and Psychiatry, 2003, Vol. 74, Issue 7. Available at: https://jnnp.bmj.com/content/74/7/837.

and the neurotransmitters have their effects. The key brain regions in our emotional network are the hippocampus, which is involved in memory; the amygdala, which produces basic emotions; the hypothalamus, which activates appetite and sexual responses; and the nucleus accumbens, which is part of our pleasure and reward system.

How are messages passed on through the maze of millions and millions of neurons in the brain? Neurosteroids, neurotransmitters and hormones are the messengers and key players in brain function. They interact with each other and are also interdependent. They help to pass or translate messages between brain cells, which can then initiate or trigger specific actions and responses. This is the brain's highway, a network of messengers, activators and responders.

The role of neurosteroids, neurotransmitters and hormones

In 1992, the French physiologist Étienne-Émile Baulieu coined the term **neurosteroids** to describe hormones that are produced in the brain (as well as in hormonal glands around the body). They interact with neurotransmitters to pass messages between brain cells, which can then alter moods and feelings. Since then, research has revealed more about the ways they are involved in mood disorders, specifically with neurotransmitters that are produced predominantly in the gut.

Neurotransmitters are the chemicals released by neurons (nerve cells) that regulate functions such as mood, sleep and appetite. They are vital for our mental and emotional health. Examples of neurotransmitters are calming GABA and feel-good serotonin. But the distinction between neurosteroids and neurotransmitters is not always that clear.

GABA, for instance, is not only a neurotransmitter, it is also the most abundant amino acid in our body and can be found specifically in grains, beans, nuts and fish. Amino acids are the building blocks for protein, which is important for muscle building and a healthy immune system. GABA's job is to damp down excessive activity in the brain, such as 'over-firing' in the amygdala, which causes anxiety, or the random firing of brain cells in epilepsy. So stimulating GABA is a way of reducing anxiety and improving sleep – and it is targeted by most sleeping pills.

Progesterone is not only a steroid hormone; it also functions as a neurotransmitter and is important for the production and action of GABA. It does this via allopregnanolone, one of the hormones that can be made from it. Progesterone and GABA track one another – when levels of one drop, so does the other. Progesterone can also be produced to a much lesser degree in the brain and plays a role in controlling anxiety and depression, as it exerts a calming effect on the nervous system. This is why it is known as 'the brain's sedative'. It also benefits the brain in a variety of other ways, such as improving thinking, damping down inflammation and helping to regrow damaged neurons.[10]

Serotonin is a neurotransmitter and the brain's feel-good chemical, helping us sleep better and feel happier. It is associated with positive mood and is targeted by antidepressant drugs. Oestrogen supports healthy serotonin levels and is essential for optimal brain function. However, this favourable connection can be upset by high levels of artificial oestrogens (xeno-oestrogens) from plastics and the like in the environment. The body responds to them as if they are real, dropping the amount of progesterone

---

10   R. D. Brinton et al., 'Progesterone receptors: form and function in brain', *Frontiers in Neuroendocrinology*, May 2008, 29(2):313–39. Available at: http://www.virginiahopkinstestkits.com/progesteronebrainresearch.html.

and leading to more intense mood swings.[11]

You may be surprised to discover that more than 90 per cent of serotonin is made in our gastrointestinal tract. This is another reason to remember to include foods in your diet that nourish the gut for optimal brain function. It may be no coincidence that the rise in obesity and poor diet has mirrored a rise in hormonally related imbalances and medical conditions.

Dopamine is an excitatory neurotransmitter in the brain that makes us feel aware, alert and focused. It can be associated with positive stress such as exercising and being in love. Drugs such as alcohol, opiates, amphetamines, nicotine and cocaine can increase dopamine. The good news is that there are lifestyle factors such as food, exercise and supplements that can have the same effect. Dairy, eggs, nuts and fish are essential, as they contain the vitamins and supplements needed for dopamine production. Oestrogen can also increase dopamine levels. It's important to get the balance right. If you have too much dopamine, you may experience anxiety or panic attacks; if it is too low, you may suffer from fatigue, sadness or lack of focus and concentration. Neurosteroids and neurotransmitters are Goldilocks chemicals – for the best effects, the amounts must be just right.

Hormones and phases of life

All is well when we are balanced hormonally and the brain is sending and receiving the correct messages. But this happy state can be disrupted at times of major hormonal change, such as

---

11   See: http://dr-lobisco.com/mood-imbalances-part-ii-the-estrogen-sero-tonin-connection/.

puberty or just before your period, after childbirth or during the perimenopause, when hormone levels, especially oestrogen, can fluctuate wildly and we lose the balance we need. There is a knock-on effect in the brain, and messages from the neurotransmitters can become scrambled.

Childhood

In early childhood, the brain continues to develop under the influence of oestrogen and testosterone. Girls' brains will develop more verbal and emotional circuits, whereas boys' will develop more neural connections for winning and exploratory behaviour.

For most girls, childhood is fairly calm. They seek social interaction and are often more talkative than boys. In general, they prefer to play with other girls, and their games and interests differ to those of boys.

Research shows evidence that the two genders begin developing different thinking skills early on. For example, three-year-old boys are able to imagine where the hands on a clock face would be to show various times – an ability known as 'mental rotation' – more accurately than girls of the same age. Pre-pubescent girls, however, are better at recalling lists of words.

These differences don't tell you anything about intelligence, but they do show that there are different patterns in ability, which are the result of the different hormone levels boys' and girls' brains are naturally exposed to.

Puberty

All this changes with the arrival of puberty, when girls are suddenly bombarded with high levels of oestrogen, progesterone and testosterone, and boys experience a flood of testosterone, pushing their level to twenty times higher than before. This hormonal differentiation will now fundamentally affect behaviour, mood, physical development, looks, desires and perception of life.

Puberty can be full of turbulent emotions for both sexes. This is the time when many young girls become obsessed with their looks. The surge of oestrogen in their brain can make them feel that being attractive to boys is the most important thing in the world. This is of course compounded by peer pressure and social media. The insurgence of fluctuating hormones and society's expectations of how they should look and behave can leave little room for individuality and getting a sense of themselves. It's a topsy-turvy time for all involved, a time when support and understanding is essential so that these young girls can become the teenagers and young adults they want to be.

CASE STUDY: JULIE

Julie is relieved and happy when at the age of fourteen she finally has her first period. Most of the girls in her class have already had theirs at least a year earlier and are interested in boys, leaving Julie feeling left out and different. She was a bit of a tomboy, who loved playing soccer and didn't really care much about her appearance. She was so pleased when she could join the club of her menstruating girlfriends.

The onset of oestrogen surging through her body and brain changes her focus dramatically. She too becomes obsessed with her looks and the ways her body is changing. She spends hours in front of the mirror trying on clothes, examining herself and playing with her hair and make-up. She wants to look beautiful and be accepted by the boys in her school. Nothing much matters except this.

Her passion for soccer and attention to schoolwork are forgotten, replaced by a drive to get boys' attention and interest. She is easily moved to tears or anger. Her parents are worried by her unreasonable behaviour and the way their little girl has become preoccupied with her appearance, her clothes and her weight.

Julie's new disposition is being sculpted by the rising levels of oestrogen, progesterone and testosterone coming in cyclical waves. From now on they will arrive monthly and vary day to day and week by week. Her brain's prefrontal cortex is becoming even more sensitive to emotional stimuli such as approval and rejection.

I'm sure many of you can relate to Julie's ups and downs. One day you feel wonderful, the next day you hate yourself. You can't bear seeing yourself in the mirror; everything and everyone irritates you, especially your family. Your body is not right, no one loves you, and with pimples erupting across your face, life just isn't worth living. But as you may remember from your own or your daughter's puberty, this phase passes.

Boys also undergo profound changes in physique and behaviour. The case history below is one that any parent of teenage boys will recognise.

CASE STUDY: BOBBY

Bobby is a delightful, inquisitive boy, the family's youngest child, who is close to his mum and loves baking with her at the weekends. But the idyll doesn't last. When he turns fourteen, his testosterone flips on and his behaviour flips with it. Adults, in particular his mother, are unbearably irritating. He stays in his room, in bed, demanding to be left alone. His voice shifts embarrassingly from squeaky to booming in response to adults asking questions. They find him almost unintelligible; he either grunts morosely or speaks fast and swallows his words.

Only his friends interest him. When his buddies come around, they disappear into his bedroom, a rank and smelly den, where his mother once found them, much to her horror, poring over pornography on his computer. He does at least blush, then shouts that she should knock before barging in.

We know that under the influence of testosterone, Bobby's brain is being rewired, stimulating the 'sexual pursuits' circuits in his hypothalamus to swell to twice the size they would be in a teenage girl.

Parents of teenagers of either sex shouldn't be surprised by the power and force of their children's fluctuating hormones, which turn them for a few years into domestic monsters. The billions of neurons that were laid down before they were born are now being stimulated into forming a mass of new connections. Whoever thought being a parent would be easy!

Reproductive years

The menstrual cycle consists of hormonal fluctuations that take place naturally from the beginning of one period to the beginning of the next menstruation. Hormones rise and fall to promote thickening of the lining of the uterus, ovulation, pregnancy or menstruation. This usually occurs every month.

THE MENSTRUAL CYCLE

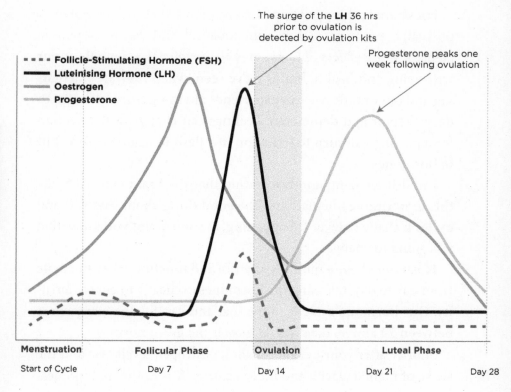

The surge of the **LH** 36 hrs prior to ovulation is detected by ovulation kits

Progesterone peaks one week following ovulation

Hormone Levels

- **- - - -** Follicle-Stimulating Hormone (FSH)
- —— Luteinising Hormone (LH)
- —— Oestrogen
- —— Progesterone

| Menstruation | Follicular Phase | Ovulation | Luteal Phase |
| Start of Cycle | Day 7 | Day 14 | Day 21 | Day 28 |

Mood changes (thoughout the cycle)

Menstruation	Follicular Phase	Ovulation	Luteal Phase
• weak immune system • dry skin • low body temperature	• increased energy • positive mood • focused	• appetite increases • increased libido	• depression • fatigue • appetite increases • increased body temperature

71

As we move into adulthood, hormones and their fluctuations will continue to affect our brain, and hence our mood, our energy, our outlook on life and our behaviour.

For women, this can happen daily, monthly, during pregnancy, postnatal, premenstrual, perimenopausal and postmenopausal. Generally, the effects of hormones are beneficial, essential for our well-being and health, but as we've seen, when they are fluctuating and out of tune, we can experience anything from 'off' days to deep despair and depression. Feelings can change fast. Affection for a partner can turn to irritation in a flash in response to a shift in hormones.

I find it amazing and fascinating that the brain can react like this to hormone fluctuations. The good thing about rhythms and cycles is that whatever is happening, at some point you know that it is going to change.

Hormones have a monthly rhythm and function. They fluctuate from day to day, releasing the hormones cyclically to enable fertility. Our hormone cycle is individual and can fluctuate anywhere between 24 and 36 days but 28 days is the given norm.

Shortly after your period finishes, oestrogen levels rise and the sense of mental clarity and focus returns. It is in the high progesterone phase, just after your periods start, that you can experience brain fog and mild cognitive decline and the end of a period is often welcomed with a sense of relief. In the first two weeks of the cycle there will be an increase in brain cell activity in the hippocampus, where memory and words are processed, and which is larger in women. Oestrogen starts to rise on day five of your cycle and peaks at ovulation, when the egg is produced ready for fertilisation. That can be any time between day 11 and day 21, but around day 14 is common.

This is when oestrogen works as a brain booster and we are

mentally at our best; we are more articulate, focused and energetic. We may feel very attractive; our libido rises, triggering a strong urge to have sex. It's obviously the time we are most likely to conceive. After that, we are back in the progesterone phase, with our brain more relaxed, which some people describe as 'fuzzy brain'.

These broad monthly rhythms are an average; you probably recognise them, but you are also likely to have your own variations. In the raised oestrogen period you can carry the world on your shoulders, your thoughts and intentions clear. But then, for no apparent reason, that changes and one morning you wake up feeling gloomy. It may be that your daily hormone level has shifted, because that in turn can influence the way you respond to stresses that normally wouldn't trouble you. Some days we can deal with stress, others not.

If hormones can have such an impact on our physical and emotional well-being in the short-term, imagine how deeply they are likely to influence us throughout the other phases of our lives.

Premenstrual syndrome

Premenstrual syndrome (PMS) is now well recognised thanks to Dr Dalton. She made the connection between hormonal imbalance and symptoms such as headaches, irritability, rage and weeping. She discovered a link between low progesterone and a number of mental and emotional problems: depression, postnatal depression, paranoid thoughts and psychosis. She even correlated menstrual cycles with antisocial behaviour, crimes committed by female prisoners and the performance of teenage girls at school during the time before their periods.

She made the connection sixty years ago, yet it is still uncommon for doctors to think of hormones as a possible underlying factor in serious psychological problems.

Dr Dalton recorded the mood swings of women in prison for violent crimes. She discovered that the acts that had put them there had often been carried out at times when they were suffering distressing menstrual symptoms. This research led to her being a key witness in several high-profile criminal cases and to establishing the legal precedent of PMS as grounds for leniency in sentencing.

One of her subjects was Nicola Owen. She was a perfectly normal child whose parents described her as 'exemplary' until the age of thirteen, when her periods began and she started to display inexplicable erratic behaviour. This included setting fire to her bedroom curtains, running away from home, being picked up by the police, shaving her head and eyebrows and slashing her fingers. At the age of seventeen she again committed arson and was immediately arrested and sent to prison. Released on bail, she took an overdose a month later, and three months after that she again set fire to her parents' house. She was returned to prison, where she slashed her wrists and tried to strangle herself with sheets tied to her window bars.

When Dr Dalton looked at Owen's records, she noticed that all these supposedly random acts of madness were in fact taking place at 28- to 30-day intervals. The dates of the insurance claims for the fires, the arrest information from the police, the date Owen's parents bought her a wig and the date her fingers were sewed up in the hospital were all linked to her menstrual cycle. Dr Dalton diagnosed her as having the newly identified disorder of premenstrual syndrome.

Nicola was released on probation and treated by Dr Dalton with progesterone supplementation. Three years later, Dr Dalton noted that she was now living a normal life. Far too many young women today who show an equally disturbed and destructive pattern of behaviour have a much less happy outcome after being treated with heavy sedative drugs.

What Nicola's case shows very clearly is that hormonal imbalance can emerge as being bigger than us, taking over our moods, actions and behaviour. It is irrational and to the outside world does not make any sense. We who suffer from hormonal imbalance do not understand what is happening. We no longer feel as if we are in control because our hormones are controlling us.

Dr Dalton's discovery of a link was a classic piece of medical sleuthing, but the events are perhaps too lurid and extreme for many to identify with. Dr Louann Brizendine described a common recurring pattern, albeit less severe, in her book *The Female Brain*. Just before the menstrual cycle ends, progesterone in the brain drops right down, leaving you feeling either hostile or hopeless. Teenagers have a more extreme reaction here because they haven't learnt how to handle it. Fortunately it doesn't take women long to realise that their moods and reactions may change just before their period. It's a time of vulnerability, and most of us learn not to act on extreme emotions because we know that it is temporary and will pass. We know that it has something to do with our hormones but we do not know why. This understanding is imperative if we are to help ourselves and take control of our well-being.

I'm sure that every menstruating woman can relate to such mood swings, whether they're the subtle swings throughout the month or the stormy fluctuations that can occur just before the period starts.

Neuropsychiatrist Dr Mona Lisa Schulz coined the phrase 'rubber band brain' to describe these cyclical changes. In her book *The New Feminine Brain*, she comments that some women are particularly sensitive to the cycling of oestrogen, progesterone and testosterone, which makes them more prone to mood, sleep and eating disorders and to suffer from premenstrual and peri-menopausal symptoms.

CASE STUDY: GLORIA

Gloria is a vivacious and ambitious 36-year-old woman who is in a steady relationship, runs her own charity shop and loves engaging with her clients and the volunteers. She knows the work she does matters and feels her life is good and rewarding.

However, she has a major, recurrent problem. The week before her period, she suffers from a huge swing in her mood. She is easily aggravated, and little things make her cry. She dreads this time of the month because she knows that she becomes unreasonable but can't control her irritability and anger. Sometimes things become so bad that she just wants to stay in bed and cry.

She is totally aware she is suffering from PMS but doesn't know how to alleviate it. She confides in her GP that she has lost control of her moods, especially her tears, and says her work doesn't give her the sense of reward it once did, and that she has begun to lose confidence in herself.

Her GP prescribes antidepressants (of course!), saying they will relieve her premenstrual symptoms and irritable moods. This is not the help that Gloria expects. In fact, being told she needs pills to cope with PMS makes her feel worse. After all, she feels fine for at least two weeks of the month and the same thing happens every month. She can see that what's needed is something that deals with the changes happening during her cycle.

So Gloria says no thanks to antidepressants and chooses to go the hormonal route to help deal with her symptoms. After a few weeks on progesterone and nutritional supplements such as magnesium, B vitamins and fish oil, her PMS symptoms are significantly reduced, and she is able to stop beating herself up about feeling bad. She begins to feel well for the whole month and her mood swings subside. She feels 'normal' again.

Antidepressants would have been a Band-Aid and would not have addressed the cause of her problem. We need to continually ask why something is happening to us in order to understand its cause and resolve it effectively.

PMS Protocol

Prescriptions of bio-identical hormones can certainly be a safe and effective way of helping with hormonal problems, but as you come to know more about your cycle, you might want to explore the possibility of reducing certain symptoms by taking supplements, following a particular diet and making some lifestyle changes that together can help with problems such as anxiety or low testosterone.

So I've put together a number of protocols containing suggestions as to how you might start. This is one for PMS that might be useful if your problem is similar to Gloria's. For more information about the effect diet can have on the state of your hormones and the healthy fats and carbohydrates you should aim to make the basis of your diet, see Chapter Four.

PMS PROTOCOL

Nutrients: vitamin B6 (B vitamins are vital for a healthy nervous system and may help with anxiety and depression), zinc (PMS sufferers given zinc supplements had lower levels of the common symptoms of depression and hostility), magnesium (essential for muscles, nerve function and sleep), L-methionine (can increase oestrogen removal in cases of oestrogen dominance), L-theanine (an amino acid found in green tea that has a calming effect), omega-3 (can improve memory, cross-talk between cells and the working of neurotransmitters; may also relieve depression), omega-6 (used by the body to create prostaglandins, which help to make hormones and boost nerve performance).

Eat more: complex carbohydrates (such as whole grains, oats, beans and brown rice). Most vegetables consist of complex carbohydrates, as do fruit and nuts. Complex carbohydrates take much longer to digest and be broken down. All carbohydrates are turned into glucose in the body. They elevate the blood sugar, which is used as energy for the body.

Reduce or avoid: sugar, caffeine, processed foods, refined carbohydrates (such as white rice, white bread, sugar, pasta and breakfast cereals; all these foods have less fibre content and nutrients), alcohol, trans/hydrogenated fats (found in biscuits and potato crisps, crackers, cakes and margarine).

Lifestyle: minimise exposure to environmental hormone disrupters such as plastic, avoid smoking, use stress management techniques to reduce stress, increase exercise.

Pregnancy

Hormonally speaking, pregnancy is one of the most extreme times in a woman's life. The combination of hormonal changes and imminent lifestyle changes can turn our moods and emotions upside down as our bodies respond to the demands of growing a new life within us. Yet often pregnant women claim they have 'never felt better'. How amazing is Mother Nature to create this paradox?

CASE STUDY: YVONNE

Yvonne is an only child and all her life she has wanted to be a mother. She loves children and became a kindergarten teacher. She enjoys being playful and enjoys the noise and laughter of the little ones, and is also able to comfort them when they are tearful or upset. She is thirty-four years old and now has her own nursery and kindergarten. She is financially fairly comfortable but has no partner, and her biological clock is ticking. Every time mothers come in with their newborns, she cradles them and is moved by their smell and their feel. Their pheromones act to strengthen her desire for a baby. She makes the decision to become a single parent.

Babies release pheromones that stimulate the hypothalamus to produce oxytocin, the hormone of intimacy, love and bonding. Of course this is what happened to Yvonne, especially when she was around babies and children, and with the increase of oxytocin her urge to become a mother and nurturer grew even more evident. The desire for a baby affects many women when they cuddle a newborn. This shows the power of hormones to make us feel and act.

During the first few weeks of pregnancy, both oestrogen and progesterone levels rise rapidly and can affect mood stability. By the sixth week, a woman's oestrogen level is approximately three times that of the highest point in the menstrual cycle, and progesterone can increase by more than forty times the level of the second half of her normal monthly cycle. All sensations can be heightened by the rise of hormones, especially taste and smell. We've all heard of food cravings in the first three months of pregnancy, or smells and tastes that one absolutely cannot tolerate and that can make one physically sick. Our brain's hunger and thirst centres are also being affected by the rising hormones.

But there are also other physical and emotional changes triggered by the rising hormones. The nipples and breasts will become tender, and there may be an overwhelming sensation of fatigue and need for sleep. This is largely the result of the pregnancy hormone progesterone, which is being produced by the placenta. This hormone can damp down the immune system during pregnancy to prevent the foetus from being rejected as foreign tissue, since half of its tissue is built by the father's DNA.

CASE STUDY: AMANDA

Amanda is in a happy relationship and gets pregnant naturally one year after starting to try for a baby. She realises very early that she is pregnant, even before missing her next period, because she suddenly develops excruciatingly tender nipples. She knows that this is one of the first symptoms of pregnancy. It isn't long before she can no longer eat her favourite pizza, as the smell and taste make her gag. Her job involves a lot of work with numbers and computers and she finds her concentration and focus flagging, especially in the afternoons, when she has an overwhelming desire to lie down and sleep. She struggles for the first three months of pregnancy and then everything settles down nicely.

By the fourth month, Amanda is no longer fatigued, and she has waves of energy and positivity. Her nausea has gone, and she can focus on work with more enthusiasm. She daydreams frequently about the growing baby inside her. Her brain has become accustomed to high levels of pregnancy hormones. When she begins to feel the first flutters of baby movements, other neuro-hormones such as oxytocin are released, and she falls more and more in love with the baby with each passing day.

Most women report feeling much better by the second trimester (three-month period) because their bodies have successfully accommodated these hormonal fluctuations. Some may even feel a sense of euphoria, and others describe how being pregnant is the best they have ever felt in their life.

As the day of delivery approaches, even more oxytocin is produced in the hypothalamus and then released into the bloodstream. This stimulates the uterine muscles to contract during labour. Relaxin (another hormone) softens the cervix and expands the pelvis, and prolactin will be stimulated and produced in excess in the pituitary gland to help breastfeeding.[12] Both oxytocin and prolactin also trigger the feelings of love and bonding between mother and baby. The father too is subjected to the onslaught of maternal and infant hormones, specifically to the pheromones the baby releases. They trigger his own hormones, and he feels love and a strong connection with the new arrival. All is well with the world!

Yes, this is the ideal situation, with mother and father's hormones and emotions in harmony. After the birth, the father's hormones become even more synchronised with the mother's if both parents are engaged in the care of their newborn. When fathers are very hands-on, their levels of the bonding hormones oxytocin and prolactin rise, while testosterone levels may drop.

This postnatal idyllic state is what nature has designed for all of us. But as we know, although nature is perfect at its origin, our

---

12   Society for Endocrinology, 'Hormones of pregnancy and labour'. Available at: http://www.yourhormones.info/topical-issues/hormones-of-pregnancy-and-labour/.

world has changed, and our environment now affects us in many ways that are completely new. Some women adjust easily, others do not.

Baby blues

If depression is something that runs in your family or something you have experienced, don't despair about handling the baby blues. There are many ways you can help yourself, such as anti-anxiety supplements, even before seeking specialist help. (See Chapter Nine.)

Pregnancy and birth can be a golden time, with the mother and father's hormones synchronising and the baby's pheromones filling them both with waves of affection and connection. But there are other natural hormonal changes going on that can introduce a darker note. During pregnancy the foetus and the placenta both release a certain amount of the stress 'fight-or-flight' hormones – cortisol and adrenaline – which produce feelings of anxiety.

During pregnancy, the massively raised levels of calming progesterone plus the extra oestrogen protects expectant mothers from these negative feelings. But when the waters break during labour, this protection is suddenly snatched away. Progesterone and oestrogen levels plummet but cortisol continues to be produced, along with oxytocin – maintaining bonding – and prolactin for breastfeeding. Cortisol without the moderating effect of progesterone can result in some new mothers becoming more stressed and anxious. About 10 per cent of women are vulnerable to developing some form of postnatal depression. In fact, there is a strong link between women who suffer from PMS and those who go on to develop postnatal depression.

But there is a bit more to this story, which shows what a complicated dance is involved in balancing hormones. Too much stress hormone during pregnancy can cause a miscarriage or developmental problems in the child later. Yet in the last few weeks of pregnancy cortisol levels can be two or three times higher than normal – an amount normally only found in people who are seriously ill. What is going on?

Interestingly, the release of cortisol from the placenta is controlled by the foetus, which means in evolutionary terms that it must be benefiting the child, but how? One idea is that cortisol influences the mother's brain so she becomes more attentive to the child. Research has found that women with higher levels of cortisol respond more strongly to a crying baby.

But scientists aren't sure yet if it is a direct effect or because cortisol pushes up oestrogen, which in turn makes the mother more responsive to the bonding effect of oxytocin. One of the ways of cutting the risk of depression after a birth is to breastfeed. Research shows that breastfeeding mothers don't respond as strongly to stressful situations as those who don't breastfeed.[13]

There is a spectrum of seriousness here, from a relatively mild case of 'baby blues', through postnatal depression, to post-partum psychosis, and they are all usually the result of the hormone roller coaster. By recognising these outcomes as a possibility, women can forearm themselves against being overwhelmed by powerful feelings.

It's normal to feel a bit tearful and wobbly, but a more prolonged bout of depression, particularly at what should be such a magical time, can often be pre-empted by understanding how and why it happens. In most cases postnatal depression can be treated

---

13   Gwen Dewar, 'Natural changes in stress hormones during pregnancy'. Available at https://www.parentingscience.com/Stress-hormones-during-pregnancy.html.

successfully with natural progesterone, with or without oestrogen, to counteract the dramatic post-partum hormonal slide.

Individual differences play a big role in all this. Some women go through life being 'hormonal', dreading the way they react to their monthly fluctuating hormones, while others never have to think about their hormones at all. They don't suffer from cyclical mood swings or headaches or food cravings or bloating or heavy periods and often don't really understand what the fuss is about.

We are all unique individuals and respond to our environment, our hormones, our stressors in our own special way. That is why there is a plethora of symptoms that we may experience when our hormones change, be it monthly, or through our reproductive years and finally when we start heading towards menopause.

Perimenopause and menopause

Menopause rarely has an obvious start date. The average age it begins is fifty-one, but it can already be under way in your early forties, long before you have had your last period and finally become menopausal. The perimenopause, when the menopause has started but before your hormones are properly switching off, can be a particularly volatile time, because just as during puberty, our hormones fluctuate inconsistently. Until this time most women can rely on their periods coming every month unless they are pregnant. Then the ovaries begin to go into a slow functional decline, and we may no longer ovulate every month. This means that we will produce less progesterone in the second part of our cycle, if any at all. It can take us a little while to really notice this subtle shift in our bodies and minds.

During the perimenopause, women can no longer rely on their hormones. Hormonal fluctuations and imbalance are on the increase and may become the norm till our periods stop permanently. Hormones can fluctuate, sometimes wildly, and can cause what I call 'Jekyll and Hyde' syndrome. Our oestrogen levels may be abnormally high or low and our progesterone levels will be in decline. We no longer feel or think like we used to. We become susceptible to sudden mood swings because our hormones are in disarray and out of balance.

CASE STUDY: SANDRA

Sandra is driving home from dropping her children off at school. It's a familiar route and she begins planning the day ahead, listing her numerous chores, calculating the best way to fit them around her part-time job as a book keeper, which she does from home. Suddenly her heart starts to race, she feels light-headed and fears she might faint at the wheel. She manages to pull over before anything dangerous happens. She sits there sweating, barely able to breathe, her heart pounding, filled with an overwhelming fear. She doesn't know what to do. She manages to call her husband, who is concerned and sends an ambulance to collect her. Sandra is diagnosed with anxiety and hyperventilation.

This describes a classic panic attack. The sense of fear can be so vivid that we respond with our fight-or-flight response – a pounding heart and a sense of doom. We may not be in any actual danger, but our judgement in these situations is often compromised. There is a disconnect between reality and our perception. A 'hormonal' panic attack commonly occurs just before a period starts, possibly because of a drop in progesterone levels. This situation is frequently exaggerated in the perimenopause. Sandra's neurotransmitter dopamine was in overdrive because she wasn't producing enough progesterone to damp down her rising sense of panic.

This transitional phase from perimenopause to menopause is different for everyone. It is a time of frequent change in hormone levels. We can no longer rely on our 28-day cycle, nor expect to continue ovulating every month and produce sufficient amounts of progesterone to balance our oestrogen fluctuations and stabilise our neurotransmitters. For some women, a tiny amount of help with balancing their hormones helps to smooth out the fluctuations and is sufficient to prevent the turmoil of hormones on the loose, allowing them to slide comfortably into being perimenopausal on the way to menopause.

Menopause

By the time we are approaching middle age, our brain has been responding for decades to the hormones that have been shaping our womanhood, our motherhood and our professional life. So what should we be doing as they start to wane during menopause? Are we really meant to live well without our life-affirming hormones?

We become postmenopausal when we have gone through the menopause – 'the change' – which is defined as beginning one year after the end of our last period. Many of my patients don't realise that once the menopause has ended, we remain postmenopausal for the rest of our lives. Some women believe that when the turbulence of the perimenopause and menopause is over, everything will be back to normal: sleep will improve, hot flushes will disappear, mood swings will lessen, memory will improve and we will be our old selves again. This may be the case for some, but not for all.

CASE STUDY: JUDITH

At fifty-four, Judith is content with her life and her new-found freedom, especially as it gives her more time to spend on herself. Her children have left home, and to combat the empty-nest syndrome, she has enrolled in a part-time course in history and anthropology at her local university. She is pleased that she is now menopausal; her periods stopped four years ago.

She is glad to be rid of them and had no symptoms afterwards. Her sleep is good, she has had no hot flushes and she doesn't understand what some of her friends are complaining about when they talk about the dreaded 'change'.

However, studying is becoming harder for Judith. She's not grasping the content properly. She feels her memory is letting her down. Instead of enjoying her new course, she's losing confidence and is now dreading going to the seminars or being asked questions on the spot. It is only when one of her friends complains about her own bad memory for names and words, and points out that this is a symptom of the menopause that Judith realises what might be happening to her.

Judith presumed that she had survived the menopause unscathed. However, the impact had taken time to show up and her memory loss and lack of concentration were most likely the result of not having enough oestrogen after it ended. Research shows that oestrogen protects the brain and that a decline may affect our mental abilities, especially memory.

All women go through these life changes, but unfortunately many do not understand what is happening to them and what they can do about it. Their GPs or specialist physicians rarely have the information, or the understanding needed to connect the dots and reveal the underlying cause.

Most women are now familiar with the idea that their hormones colour their reality, but even so, many of us still don't fully grasp what a fundamental impact this has and how profoundly this new-found knowledge can help us live life to the full.

Our hormones affect us through their subtle daily shifts, more strongly through the monthly cycle and then through the massive hormonal emotional swings during pregnancy or perimenopause. Of course, the impact on everyone is not always dramatic. Some of us may be hurled through our normal environment like a dinghy in a stormy sea; others meet the changes as though they were rowing gently across a placid lake.

We are fortunate today that we know about the importance of hormones for our brain chemistry and for the long-term effects they have on our physical and mental health. We should take advantage of this and be focused on hormone balancing. The time for bio-identical hormone replacement therapy has come.

But even bio-identical hormones don't work in a vacuum. Food, supplements, lifestyle, exercise and mindfulness all play a part in helping you to feel better, become calmer and bring the joy back into your life. So before I tell you more about the various ways specific hormones can help, read the next chapter about some of the things we can all do to help ourselves.

SUMMARY OF KEY POINTS

- Our hormonal rhythms should be a cause for celebration.
- Hormonal influences on our brains start when we're in the womb.
- Oestrogen and progesterone have very different effects on the developing brain.
- The brain has a network of areas that work together to control emotions.
- Oestrogen can make men weep and women forgetful.
- There is a delicate dance between our hormones and the brain's messengers – the neurotransmitters.
- Neurotransmitters enable signals to pass from one neuron to a target cell.
- Hormones have different effects on us through our life cycle, from childhood, through the turbulence of puberty and the fluctuations during a monthly cycle, to pregnancy, birth, peri-menopause and the menopause.
- Pre-menstrual syndrome – this can be so serious for some women that experts have been able to link female crime and that time of the month.
- There are ways to help with hormonal imbalances such as PMS by looking at supplements, food and lifestyle.
- In the perimenopause and menopause, hormones become unreliable, and for some women this causes mood swings and physical symptoms. There are ways to help with a food and lifestyle protocol.
- Effective hormone replacement *is* available.

CHAPTER FOUR

HOW FOOD AND DIET AFFECT MOODS AND BEHAVIOUR

● ● ● ●

So far we have talked about the way our hormone levels can fluctuate and change over the years, and how this can bring both blissful feelings and despair. A sensible response to signs that our hormones are out of balance is to find out what is missing and offer bio-identical replacements. Our hormones are sensitive to the changes that come with age and to the stresses that are a normal part of living. But there is something else that may have a major impact on how your hormones behave – what you eat.

Given the huge range of bodily functions affected by hormones, including blood sugar balance, blood pressure, energy levels, kidney function, sleep patterns and appetite, you might think they would be one of the first things to check when you are complaining of typical symptoms of a hormone problem. These can include fatigue, headaches, digestive complaints, poor sleeping, easy weight gain, increased signs of ageing, depression, anxiety and decreased sexual desire.

But just as the medical profession hasn't caught up with the potential for treating mental disorders with replacement bioidentical hormones, so diet as a factor in hormone disruption is also not really on their radar. A sensible starting point for a hormone-friendly diet would be to get enough dark leafy greens, a 'rainbow' of brightly coloured vegetables, a good amount of protein and plenty of water.

But this doesn't tell you anything about how much fat and how many carbs you need, or whether proteins from meat or vegetables are better, or provide advice on other current controversies such as a low-carb vs a vegetarian diet.

There isn't a diet for everyone

The idea that there is one diet that fits everyone is not really plausible any more, as Professor Tim Spector pointed out recently.[1] He has found that something as simple as the amount your blood sugar level is raised by eating a carbohydrate can vary enormously. One person can have blood sugar spikes after a bowl of pasta but sees no rise with grapes; another can have the opposite response to the same foods. This can have a knock-on effect on hormones, because they are affected by how many carbs you are eating.

As for our vastly complicated microbiome – the three-pound colony of trillions of bacteria in our gut – the way that responds to diet seems to be equally individual. Every day brings new reports of the role it plays in the immune system, our emotional responses and, yes, the production of hormones – oestrogen in particular.

---

1   Tim Spector, 'Butter or margarine? Food religion challenged', *British Medical Journal, December 2018*. Available at:
https://blogs.bmj.com/bmj/2018/12/17/tim-spector-butter-or-margarine-food-religion-challenged/?utm_campaign=shareaholic&utm_medium=twitter&utm_source=socialnetwork.

Fat is no longer the demon

For decades we were told that keeping fat intake low was the key to weight loss, protection against heart disease and general health. Now it's clear that any weight you do lose on a low-fat calorie-controlled diet is very likely to go back on, and that this diet has little measurable impact on heart health. Constant promotion of the diet has, however, led to a significant increase in the amount of sugar in processed foods, with subsequent effects on the incidence of obesity and diabetes.

Even less hormonally beneficial has been the impact of the low-fat theory on keeping cholesterol low. The flaws in the cholesterol hypothesis have been the subject of many books and research papers; Dr Malcolm Kendrick's *The Great Cholesterol Con* is particularly accessible.[2] Cholesterol is vital for hormonal regulation because it is the raw material the body uses to make hormones such as oestrogen, testosterone and progesterone.

So there is now a growing number of people who no longer worry about fat in their diet (although vegetarians and especially vegans avoid animal fats and point to the risks of eating meat), and cutting sugar intake has become official policy instead. Obesity has a knock-on effect on hormones, as the stored fat can push your oestrogen levels unhealthily high.

---

2   Dr Malcolm Kendrick, *The Great Cholesterol Con: the truth about what really causes heart disease and how to avoid it,* John Blake, 2007.

Get enough, but not too much, protein

Protein is the other food group that is vital for a favourable hormone balance, which is why protein-rich foods as well as supplements of the amino acids that build proteins are sometimes known as 'mood foods'. They can provide the building blocks for the neurotransmitters we met in Chapter Three, such as serotonin and dopamine, which trigger moods and emotional responses. The amino acid tryptophan is an example. It's found in foods such as nuts, red meat, fish, beans and eggs, and is used by the body to make feel-good serotonin, which can be switched on by oestrogen. It can also be taken as a supplement, often with another amino acid, 5-HTP.

The most familiar sources of the essential amino acids are the proteins found in organic meats, cheese, eggs, fish, poultry and game; most of them are available in supplement form too. However, essential amino acids are also available from vegetarian sources.

Eating to feed the brain is a good idea

The idea that food can play a role in treating mental disorders seems like common sense: if your brain is deprived of the right nutrition, it won't function properly. But it's only recently that this has been taken up by psychiatrists. There is a flourishing new field of nutritional psychiatry exploring the many correlations between the way we feel, the way we behave and the way we eat.

A paper published recently[3] sets out the basic idea, looking at the

---

3   Wolfgang Marx, 'Nutritional psychiatry: the present state of the evidence', *Proceedings of the Nutrition Society,* November 2017, Vol. 76, Issue 4, pp.427–36.

various damaging processes that could be going on in the brain, such as inflammation, too many free radicals (oxidative stress) and a poorly functioning gut microbiome. One of the most disastrous is a breakdown in the system for growing new brain cells (neuro-plasticity), which is vital because the brain is constantly reorganising itself and needs to build new neurons. This plasticity is also important for keeping hormone levels balanced,[4] as neurosynaptic plasticity is essential for the remodelling of neurosecretory neurons in the hypothalamus that may participate in the regulation of hormonal release. Among the supplements that look promising for reversing some of these functional failures are omega-3 fatty acids, the B vitamin folate, and a synthetic version of a natural chemical known as SAMe (S-Adenosyl methionine), which has been found to improve symptoms of depression and schizophrenia.

Carbohydrates and glucose

All this changes our idea of what makes up a healthy diet – fats back in favour, sugar out in the cold – and raises the question of how much carbohydrate we should be eating for hormone health. The brain certainly needs carbohydrates, because it is the most energy-demanding organ in the body, and glucose (sugar), made when the body breaks down carbs, is a major source of its energy. Glucose is needed to provide the energy for making the neurotransmitters discussed in Chapter Three and it supplies at least 50 per cent of the energy our brain demands just to maintain day-to-day functions.

---

4   Luis Miguel García-Segura, *Hormones and Brain Plasticity*, Oxford Scholarship Online, 2009.

But carbohydrates are not only important as an energy source; they also play an additional role in how we feel, as they make it easier to absorb the amino acids we need to produce the all-important brain chemical serotonin. That's why we might well regard a plate of pasta as comfort food; we may feel calmer and more relaxed after eating it.

Get your carbs complex, not simple

Carbohydrates are made up of the sugars, starches and fibres found in fruits, grains, vegetables and milk products. They come in two forms – simple and complex. The simple, or refined, ones are made up of just a few sugar molecules and are digested and absorbed much more rapidly into the bloodstream. You find them in the likes of bread, cake, flour, rice, fizzy drinks and sweets. They will give you a short-term high or 'sugar hit', which will briefly push your blood glucose level up. Straight afterwards you may feel tired and fuzzy, and will soon feel hungry again. They should be eaten very sparingly, if at all.

Complex carbohydrates are made up of hundreds of sugar molecules, fibre starches and nutrients. They are found in foods such as fruit and vegetables, whole grains and legumes (beans). The sugars they contain are absorbed and digested much more gradually than simple carbs, so they provide the brain with a consistent slow-release supply of energy and nutrients. This keeps us clearly focused and boosts brain function.

Starches make up the biggest part of complex carbohydrates and have several beneficial effects on our system. They improve insulin sensitivity and reduce blood sugar levels, as well as providing an important food source for the bacteria in our microbiome, which use them to make short-chain fatty acids (SCFAs) such as butyrate, needed to create cholesterol, which in turn is the raw material for all the steroid hormones such as oestrogen, progesterone and testosterone. So whole foods – and a minimum of processed ones – that come with slow-release starches and fibre are a good starting place for a hormone-healthy diet.

There's evidence that testosterone benefits from a good supply of carbohydrates, because when glucose can't get into cells because of insulin resistance – when your blood sugar is too high – the total amount of testosterone drops.[5] On the other hand, combining a high level of carbs with intensive exercise pushes up the amount of accessible testosterone.

A low-carbohydrate diet and your hormones

Until recently, the decades-old advice was that starchy carbohydrates should make up at least half of your food intake. This means that we should all be aiming for around 200 to 250 grams of carbs a day and eat considerably less fat. But increasing evidence of the safety and benefits of fat has encouraged many to go on low-carb ketogenic diets that are the opposite of this advice – high in fat and low in carbohydrates, with a number of significant health benefits.[6]

The ketogenic diet recommends that you drastically cut your carbohydrate intake to between 20 and 50 grams a day and replace the missing calories with fat. This avoids the constant hunger that made the calorie-controlled, low-fat diet a challenge. The ketogenic

---

5   R. Pasquali et al., 'Insulin regulates testosterone and sex hormone-binding globulin concentrations in adult normal weight and obese men', *Journal of Clinical Endocrinology & Metabolism*, 1995, 80(2):654–8.
6   Jerome Burne and Patrick Holford, *The Hybrid Diet*, Little Brown, 2019.

diet has attracted a lot of attention for weight loss and as a treatment for diabetes.[7] But it also offers a radical new way of affecting brain control of hormones.

Ketones: how your brain works without glucose

On the ketogenic diet, the body responds to the rapid drop in carbohydrates by using the fat released from storage to make small, dense molecules called ketones that can be used for energy by the brain and muscles. We all know that the brain needs lots of glucose for energy. What's less well known is that it can't use fat. This is where ketones come in. They are made in the liver from fat and have allowed us to survive times of famine with a fully functioning brain.

So what are the effects of the ketone diet on hormone production? Does it have any particular benefits or risks? Sharply cutting back on carbohydrates – going from around 200 grams a day to 20 or 30 grams – is a shock to the system, which responds as if there were a famine on the way and starts making various metabolic changes to handle it.

The most immediate effect of a severe lack of carbohydrates is that your blood glucose – made from carbs – starts dropping, quickly followed by the level of the hormone insulin in your blood.

This is very good news if you have a common condition known as insulin resistance, which often goes hand in hand with obesity and diabetes. Insulin resistance, and its opposite, insulin sensi-

---

7   Sarah J. Hallberg et al., 'Effectiveness and Safety of a Novel Care Model for the Management of Type 2 Diabetes at 1 Year: An Open-Label, Non-Randomized, Controlled Study', *Diabetes Therapy*, 2018, 9:583–612. Available at: https://doi.org/10.1007/s13300-018-0373-9.

tivity, has a profound effect on sex hormone balance. When your body is sensitive to insulin, levels of testosterone, progesterone and oestradiol in both men and women are more likely to remain at the right level.[8] The damaging effects of insulin resistance include sugar cravings and weight gain.

So starting on the ketogenic diet significantly improves insulin sensitivity, which pushes oestrogen, progesterone and testosterone back up. The ketogenic diet also improves the regularity of ovulation and menstruation and is generally good for women's health. It can certainly be beneficial if you are overweight and sedentary, with chronic metabolic problems.

Besides the considerable benefit of improved insulin sensitivity and making weight loss easier, the diet means that your brain is running on ketones. Some people claim that this makes them clear-headed and gives them greater mental clarity; there is certainly evidence that ketones can protect brain cells.

The downside to ketones

Some people, however, find the changes the diet requires stressful to begin with, although the hunger that is part of a low-fat calorie-controlled diet is not a problem because you are replacing the lost carbohydrates with fat, which in turn increases production of the hormone leptin, which reduces hunger.

But you do have to stop eating many of the familiar and favourite carbohydrate foods – bread, rice, root vegetables – which you may

---

8　A. J. M. Al-Fartosy and I. M. Mohammed, 'Biochemical Study of the Effects of Insulin Resistance on Sex Hormones in Men and Women Type-2 Diabetic Patients', *Advances in Biochemistry*, October 2017, Vol. 5, Issue 5, pp.79–88. Available at: http://www.sciencepublishinggroup.com/journal/paperinfo?journalid=110&doi=10.11648/j.ab.20170505.11.

find hard. They are replaced with meat, fish, dairy, and vegetables high in fat such as avocado.

People on the diet may take some time to discover the amounts of fat and carbs that work best for them. Some are nervous of eating too much fat after years of being told that it is dangerous, but it can quickly have a beneficial effect. One study found that eating just 5 per cent more fat than usual increased oestrogen and DHEA levels by 12 per cent in women after menopause.[9]

Lowering carbohydrates too far can reduce thyroid hormone production in some people (women in particular), as the thyroid gland is particularly sensitive to nutritional deficiencies; this may also lower progesterone. The problem is usually cured by upping the carb intake to at least 50 grams, providing you are getting the other nutritional factors you need – adequate protein, along with the vitamins A, B2 and B12, C and D, plus the minerals magnesium, zinc and iodine.

One way of regulating your carb intake until you get it right is by carb cycling – keeping it low for five days of the week and then having rather more at the weekend. Fewer carbs sharpens up your insulin sensitivity, which means you produce more of a compound called glycogen, made from carbs, that helps you burn fat.

---

9   C. Nagata et al., 'Fat intake is associated with serum estrogen and androgen concentrations in postmenopausal Japanese women', *Journal of Nutrition*, December 2005, 135(12):2862–5. Available at: https://www.ncbi.nlm.nih.gov/pubmed/16317133.

Proteins: bricks and mortar for building the body and brain

Most of your body – skin, organs, eyes, muscles – is made up of protein, and the building blocks of protein are amino acids. There are nine essential amino acids; essential here means that they can't be made by the body, so we have to get them from our diet. These are the ones we are concentrating on. Among the best sources are meat, fish, dairy, eggs, nuts and seeds.

Just as some hormones can act as the raw material for others – testosterone to make oestrogen, for instance – so the essential amino acids can form part of the production chain to make others. For instance, L-phenylalanine (best source, among many: egg whites) is converted into L-tyrosine, which can then either be made into the thyroid hormones or into L-dopa in the brain, which is then converted into the pleasure brain chemical dopamine. L-tyrosine, found in meat, fish, eggs and some vegetables, is also available as a supplement and is said to be helpful for alertness, memory and handling stress.

But to turn the amino acids into proteins or to turn one hormone into another, you also need the right minerals and vitamins. Some proteins cannot be made without B vitamins, for instance, while to make the thyroid hormone T4, your body needs iodine, zinc and selenium. Providing you are eating reasonably healthily, you can normally get both the essential amino acids and the minerals and vitamins from your diet. But for all sorts of reasons, you may not be able to get all you need. Choosing the most effective combination is an expert job, and taking advice from a nutritionist is a good idea. That way you can work out exactly what you are missing. But you can also make sure you eat a range of foods that supply all the essential amino acids. For non-vegetarians, the best sources are organic meats, cheese, eggs, fish, poultry and game.

There are vegetarian amino acid sources, but you do need to pay more attention if you are going to get all the essentials. Soy, quinoa and buckwheat are plant-based foods that contain all nine essential amino acids. Many other plant foods, such as beans and nuts, contain a range of amino acids but miss one or two, so you need to make sure you eat a variety of different plant protein sources every day.

GABA is the only amino acid that is also a neurotransmitter. It has a calming effect on the brain as it inhibits the actions of dopamine and norepinephrine, which have an excitatory effect. People who have symptoms of low GABA, such as irritability, anxiety, insomnia and poor mental focus, can improve them by eating foods that contain GABA, or supplement with L-theanine, which we find in green tea. It is well-known that although green tea contains caffeine, we still experience a sense of calm when we drink it because the theanine helps in the formation of GABA. The main source of GABA supplements are fermented foods such as kefir, miso, sauerkraut, tempeh and yogurt.

Fats: no longer bad, and good for the brain

We have been warned against eating too much fat for decades, so it's an interesting fact that our brain is mainly made up of fats and that they are crucial for optimal brain function and development. Essential fatty acids such as omega-3 and omega-6 are needed to build the cell walls of billions of nerve cells that are responsible for constructing and releasing the neurotransmitters in our brain. These fats are also important for mood, concentration, memory, learning and intelligence. Those following the long-standing advice to eat a low-fat diet may well find it hard to obtain enough fat to absorb fat-soluble vitamins A, D and E. This is not a problem on the low-carb diet mentioned earlier.

Omega-3 fats come from cold-water fish such as salmon and mackerel, but they originate from the algae that some fish feed on, which can provide a vegetarian source. An inadequate supply of essential omega-3 fatty acids may be a factor in developing depression. Another benefit of omega-3 is that it allows you to synthesise protein more effectively.[10]

Omega-6 essential fatty acid (linoleic acid) comes from flax-seed, pumpkin and sunflower seeds. Grapeseed oil, evening primrose oil and borage oil are all good sources of omega-6 and should be included in the food you eat.

Ideally you should aim to eat omegas-3 and 6 in a 1:2 ratio, but if you are following a standard Western diet, that ratio is more likely to be 1:15. One way of reducing your omega-6 intake is to avoid industrially produced vegetable oils and to supplement 3 to 4 grams daily of omega-3 and 1 to 2 grams of whole-food-based omega-6 linoleic acid.

There is evidence that different types of fat can affect the production of testosterone. One study found that those eating a high level of saturated fatty acids (SFAs), found in foods such as coconut oil and fatty meat, or monounsaturated fatty acids (MUFAs), found in avocado, olive oil and goose fat, produced more testosterone, while those getting polyunsaturated fatty acids (PUFAs),

---

10 G. I. Smith et al., 'Dietary omega-3 fatty acid supplementation increases the rate of muscle protein synthesis in older adults: a randomized controlled trial', *American Journal of Clinical Nutrition,* February 2011, 93(2):402–12. Available at: doi: 10.3945/ajcn.110.005611.

commonly found in industrial vegetable oils, had a drop in testosterone production.[11]

Cholesterol: vital for making hormones

The long-running demonisation of fat is closely tied up with the campaign to keep lowering the official safe level of the fatty substance cholesterol. Many experts now recognise that there is a contradiction between the warnings about the dangers of high cholesterol and the many important roles that it plays in the body. Besides being the raw material for the hormones active in the brain, it is also an essential element in the construction of cell walls and is vital for communication between brain cells.

Without cholesterol, the junctions (synapses) between nerves would fail to pass on messages. The membranes at these junctions are lined with cholesterol-rich membranes that release various neurotransmitters such as serotonin, GABA and dopamine. Cholesterol also provides the crucial insulation around nerves (myelin sheath), transmitting electrical impulses, and helps with the digestion of fat-soluble vitamins A, D, E and K. So it is not surprising that the brain contains about 25 per cent of all the cholesterol found in the body. In fact, so essential is it that the brain makes its own supply.

If the brain is low on cholesterol, or starved of the right fats, the membranes at the junctions will not be able to function properly. Brain chemistry will be disturbed, as will mood and behaviour. The fact that high cholesterol levels are associated with better memory and that low levels have been associated with depression shows just how essential it is.

---

11   Jeff S. Volek et al., 'Testosterone and cortisol in relationship to dietary nutrients and resistance exercise', *Journal of Applied Physiology*, January 1997, 82(1):49–54. Available at: http://jap.physiology.org/content/82/1/49.

So how can it be, you may now be asking, that the medical community continues to ramp up its 'war on cholesterol' and is in favour of prescribing prophylactic cholesterol-lowering drugs (statins) to everyone over the age of fifty? This is too big a topic to include in this book, but there is a debate going back at least a decade between those supporting the official line and a loose network of clinicians and researchers who have produced careful research challenging it.

The microbiome: a major player in the brain

So we've learnt that two of the compounds that play major roles in affecting moods and emotions in the brain – hormones and cholesterol – are so important that the brain makes them on site. But there is another player pulling strings that has been almost entirely ignored until very recently: the microbiome, that complex colony of billions of bacteria living in our gut. Given the attention I've paid to the role of the neurotransmitter serotonin in the brain, it may come as a surprise to learn that 95 per cent of your serotonin, along with 60–80 per cent of your immune system, is found in your gut.

In fact, the gut has a specific name for its own nervous system, the enteric nervous system, and its immune system, the GALT-gut associated lymphoid tissue. This enteric nervous system interacts with many different enzymes and hormones (leptin, ghrelin, insulin) to send feedback to the brain.

Sometimes described as our second brain, the gut is lined with millions of nerve cells and produces the neurotransmitters that are essential for our brain chemistry. Who hasn't felt tummy rumblings or cramping or flutters when anxious or worried? Our gut will respond to our emotions because of these millions of neurons and the neural pathways between our intestines and the brain.

It therefore makes sense that we need to feed our gut and thus ourselves with the best foods. The gut directly affects our emotions and behaviour. It is the home of serotonin production. We need the right environment to benefit from our foods. Digestion is highly dependent on the billions of 'good' bacteria living in a healthy gastrointestinal tract. These bacteria protect our gut and help us absorb the nutrients we need, and also set up the nerves linking the guts with the brain.

What this means is that the way we feed the gut is going to have effects throughout the body. Several studies have found that the vegetarian DASH (dietary approaches to stop hypertension) diet – whole grains, fruit and vegetables – is linked with lower rates of depression;[12] other studies of diets with lots of fruit and vegetables and not much meat or dairy found the same effect. This could be because the fibres in a plant-based diet feed the bacteria in the gut, which can reduce the inflammation in the brain linked with depression.

Supplements for brain chemistry, mood and energy

Depending on how good your diet is, you may need to add some vitamins and minerals, both for general health and to make sure you have enough to keep your hormones in the right balance. You may already have noticed the protocol in Chapter Three – advice

---

12 Olga Khazan, 'The Diet that Might Cure Depression', *The Atlantic*, 29 March 2018.

on the best combinations of supplements, foods and lifestyle changes to help to keep your hormones running smoothly just before your periods. Here is one for the arrival of the menopause.

PERIMENOPAUSE PROTOCOL

Nutrients: Vitamin B6 and B12 (B vitamins are vital for a healthy nervous system and may help with anxiety and depression), zinc (PMS sufferers given zinc supplements had lower levels of the common symptoms of depression and hostility), magnesium (essential for muscles, nerve function and sleep), L-methionine (can increase oestrogen removal in cases of oestrogen dominance), L-theanine (an amino acid found in green tea that has a calming effect), omega-3 (can improve memory, cross-talk between cells and the working of neurotransmitters; may also relieve depression), omega-6 (used by the body to make prostaglandins, which help to make hormones and boost nerve performance).

Eat more: complex carbohydrates, vegetables, fruit, nuts, oily fish, whole grains, purified water.

Reduce or avoid: sugar, caffeine, processed foods, refined carbohydrates, alcohol, trans/hydrogenated fats.

Lifestyle: minimise exposure to environmental hormone disrupters such as plastic, avoid smoking, use stress management techniques to reduce stress, increase exercise.

'Let food be thy medicine and medicine thy food'

This famous quote came from Hippocrates over 2500 years ago! When we eat healthy, organic unprocessed food we feel well and energised. Unadulterated foods contain the most minerals and vitamins which we need to support all our bodily functions, including brain function, physical activity and sleep. Hippocrates was right. When we eat well, we live well and healthily. Here is a short list of food groups, vitamins, minerals and herbs we should consider having in our diet.

Carbohydrates

These provide us with energy that is more instant and readily available than the supply we get from fat. You need complex carbs that are slowly absorbed.

These are some good sources:

- oatmeal
- brown rice
- sweet potato and yams
- multigrain cereal (barley, oats and rye)
- white potato with skins
- wholewheat bread
- wholewheat pasta
- beans and lentils
- couscous
- quinoa
- beets

- butternut squash
- pumpkin

It is also helpful to eat vegetables that are rich in the vital vitamins and contain important minerals such as potassium, calcium, phosphorus, magnesium, zinc, copper, manganese, selenium and chromium.

These are some good sources:

- broccoli
- kale
- asparagus
- spinach
- salad greens
- tomatoes
- peppers
- onion
- mushrooms
- cucumber
- courgettes
- carrots
- green beans
- peas
- cauliflower

Fats

These are a source and storage box of energy. Some contain essential fatty acids that the body cannot make. They are also the building blocks of both the membrane that surrounds every cell and the steroid hormones. A good supply is needed for you to absorb the fat-soluble vitamins E, D and K.

These are some healthy sources:

- flaxseed/linseed
- almonds
- olive oil
- avocado
- walnuts
- virgin coconut oil
- wild salmon
- peanuts
- ghee (clarified butter)
- peanut oil
- olives
- hemp seed oil
- pecan
- cashews
- dark chocolate

Protein

Protein is needed for the repair, growth and maintenance of the body's tissues and cells. It maintains muscles, bones and organs.

These are some good sources:

- eggs
- organic poultry
- turkey breast
- wild salmon
- tuna

- nuts (walnuts, almonds, pecans)
- pumpkin
- sesame seeds
- organic beef
- tofu
- Greek yoghurt
- cod
- rainbow trout

Vitamin and minerals

Vitamin and mineral deficiencies need treating for hormone health.

B vitamins are vital for stress tolerance as well as being essential for proper nervous system function. B vitamin deficiencies are often associated with anxiety and nervous disorders.

Vitamin E may be beneficial in nervousness and depression.

Vitamin D (cholecalciferol) is the only vitamin that is actually a hormone. It is produced in the skin from 7-dehydrocholesterol when it is exposed to UVB (ultraviolet B rays) in sunlight. Vitamin D deficiency may be a contributor to depressive symptoms that occur during wintertime, when there is relatively little sunshine. This may affect serotonin levels in the brain.

Magnesium is a smooth muscle relaxant and has a calming effect on nerves. It is needed to balance neurotransmitters in the brain to alleviate mood swings.

Calcium together with magnesium is needed for the proper function of muscles and nerves. Deficiencies in these minerals may lead to irritability, tension and insomnia.

Zinc is an essential trace element for healthy brain function.

Selenium is an important micronutrient for the brain and thyroid function.

SAMe is a synthetic form of a compound made naturally in the body that is available as a supplement. It has been found to be helpful for depression and for improving mood and immune function, as well as to control pain.

Herbs

There are a number of herbs that have been found to encourage the healthy functioning of various hormones and neurotransmitters.

Rhodiola, also known as arctic or golden root, helps balance cortisol levels. It can enhance the transport into the brain of serotonin precursors such as tryptophan and 5-HTP. This in turn increases serotonin activity in the brain.

Siberian ginseng increases our tolerance and response to stress, be it mental, physical or environmental. It can help in the production and regulation of adrenal gland hormones. It supports adrenal function, which is very important for those suffering from chronic stress.

Ginkgo biloba (maidenhair tree) is beneficial in improving memory and cognitive function, boosting mood and increasing energy. It works by enhancing the brain's microcirculation and utilising glucose and oxygen in the brain cells.

Dong quai (*Angelica sinensis*) is also known as 'female ginseng'. It is one of the most used female tonics worldwide and is commonly used for menopausal symptoms. Dong quai may have an oestrogen-regulating effect and can relieve hot flushes, palpitations and irritability.

St John's wort (*Hypericum perforatum*) has been scientifically shown to relieve mild to moderate depression. It may also improve mood swings, relieve anxiety and reduce symptoms of premenstrual tension.

Feverfew is a flowering plant from the daisy family. Ingesting feverfew can reduce the frequency of migraine headaches and symptoms, including pain, nausea, vomiting and sensitivity to light and noise.

Black cohosh is a natural sedative for people who suffer from chronic anxiety, stress, insomnia or non-restful sleep.

Green tea contains an amino acid that has been linked with a range of benefits such as reducing anxiety, improving sleep, lowering stress and helping with depression.

SUMMARY OF KEY POINTS

- This chapter covers the basics of the hormone-friendly diet, but is not 'one-size-fits-all'.
- The low-fat diet is not hormone friendly.
- Protein: get enough but not too much.
- Psychiatrists have started paying attention to food for the brain.
- Complex carbohydrates feed the brain.

- Good carbs help with testosterone levels.
- The low-carb diet has a big affect on your hormones.
- Ketones let your brain work without glucose. They can help with hormone balance, but the ketonic diet should be followed with care.
- Proteins: where meat eaters and vegetarians can find the essential amino acids.
- Vitamins and minerals can help your brain and its hormone needs.
- Fats containing omega-3 and omega-6 have big benefits.
- Cholesterol is vital for your hormones, but does it really harm the heart?
- The microbiome is the secret controller of your hormones and you can eat to feed it.
- PMS protocol: diet and lifestyle changes can help.
- Certain vitamins, minerals and herbs can help your hormones.

CHAPTER FIVE

HORMONES ON THE LOOSE

● ● ● ●

One of the constant themes of this book is that female hormones are linked with depression. Women who suffer from PMS or are menopausal who complain of feeling low or irritable or tired are routinely prescribed antidepressants. There are stacks of research papers making claims such as that women are twice as likely to suffer from depression, anxiety and other mood disorders as men.

A similar message comes from the World Health Organization, which concludes that the 'female gender is a significant predictor of being prescribed mood altering psychotropic drugs', and that 'depression is not only the most common women's mental health problem but is more persistent in women than men'.[1]

This is quite an indictment, and certainly a handicap for women to carry with them on their journey to a healthy, fulfilled life. Why should being female mean that many of us may need to take mind-altering drugs, specifically antidepressants? Being female is not a medical condition; puberty, pregnancy and menopause are not generally medical conditions, so why does being a woman carry with it such an apparent blight on our mental

---

1   https://www.who.int/mental_health/media/en/242.pdf

well-being? Why is depression generally twice as common in women as in men?

It is certainly true, as we've seen in earlier chapters, that changes in our hormones affect our emotions. But at this point we find ourselves in a catch-22. Linking hormones with feeling weepy or anxious or angry has long been an excuse for discrimination. We are unreliable, unstable because of our hormones, so we are less likely to be able to handle demanding jobs. But denying the link makes it much harder to get the replacement and balancing of hormones that I and thousands of my patients know to be effective.

Unfortunately, doctors are stuck in a similar bind. There is plenty of scientific research showing a link between our hormones and our emotions. But the explanation for why can be very vague. One doctor I came across said that it was due to 'the cyclical mix of hormones that flows through their neural pathway'. Not very helpful if you want to know how to treat patients. So rather than trying to change the underlying cause, most doctors can only apply the equivalent of a sticking plaster by prescribing antidepressants.

Pregnancy: hit by a hormone crash

What is absolutely in no doubt is the power of hormones to drive women to do the most desperate and dreadful things. As we've seen, this was clearly demonstrated sixty years ago by Dr Dalton, who found that the emotional distress created by hormones every month drove some women to acts that landed them in prison.

The monthly hormonal cycle drove the poet Sylvia Plath to regular emotional outbursts and self-harming actions. Hormones can all too easily put you on the path of depression, violence and suicide. But with proper treatment, that misery can very often be prevented or alleviated. One reason why women are at greater risk of depression is because they are not getting effective treatment when their risk rises.

One of the most dramatic and shocking cases I have encountered involved a patient of mine called Lucy, who was driven to violent action very soon after she had given birth; a time of great hormonal change.

CASE STUDY: LUCY

Lucy was twenty-six when she arrived in my clinic with her husband Mike. She seemed very calm and told me that 'at the moment' she was in a 'good space'. It quickly became clear, however, that for the last three years she had been having a very difficult time.

Lucy had a three-year-old son, but the birth had been long and painful and afterwards she was exhausted. When the midwife placed the baby in her arms, she was overwhelmed with a sense of fear and anxiety. Both she and her husband felt the enormity of the responsibility they were facing and were frightened. Although Lucy was exhausted, she couldn't sleep. When the nurse gave her the baby to cuddle, she felt inadequate and pushed him away.

On discharge day, while Mike was finalising the paperwork, Lucy jumped out of the first-floor window of her hospital room with the baby in her arms. It was an almost unimaginably awful event.

To the relief of all, the baby wasn't hurt and Lucy survived with minor injuries. However, she was sectioned and sent to a psychiatric ward, where she remained for three months, and was prescribed antidepressants and sedatives. She also received a lot of cognitive behavioural therapy (CBT). What Lucy did was inexplicable to herself and to her family, but she had a good support network to help her find her way back into a 'normal' life.

She told me, however, that she had never felt like her old self again. During the previous three years she had tried many antidepressants, but none seemed to help with her underlying anxiety, though she was now a very attentive mother and Mike a hands-on father. She had come to me on the advice of a psychotherapist she was seeing, who was happy for her to seek a hormonal solution for her continuing symptoms.

Blood tests showed that Lucy had high oestrogen levels and very low progesterone. I prescribed progesterone cream to be taken mornings and evenings, and she and Mike couldn't believe the effect. For the first time in three years, Lucy felt relaxed. She'd never realised how tense and highly strung she had been all that time. With the help of Mike and her therapist and the progesterone treatment, she learnt to live with her guilt.

I was delighted with the result but felt it was tragic that Lucy had had to wait so long to get some effective treatment. It was obvious that part of her crisis was due to the dramatic drop in calming progesterone. Her pregnancy had been unremarkable. There had been no telltale signs that she was at risk of such a severe and drastic reaction. She had had no history of depression or anxiety or other mental health issues, and no record of PMS. The lack of any warning makes it almost certain that her crisis was directly due to the changes in her hormones. It's true that family and professional support had helped with her recovery, but it could have happened much more quickly and easily if her system had been back up and running on the missing hormones right away.

Although replacing her missing progesterone was the first priority, Lucy might also have benefited from one of the food and lifestyle *protocols developed specifically to address anxiety, something she continued to suffer from for three years after the birth despite being prescribed a variety of antidepressants.*

ANXIETY PROTOCOL

Nutrients: magnesium (essential for muscles, nerve function and sleep), flaxseed oil, also known as hemp oil (high in the plant version of omega-3 fats; some studies finds it reduces inflammation), rhodiola extract, also known as arctic or golden root (used in traditional medicine to improve mood and reduce the effect of stress), L-theanine (an amino acid found in green tea that has a calming effect).

Eat more: complex carbohydrates, vegetables (especially dark leafy greens), fruit, nuts and seeds, oily fish, whole grains.

Reduce or avoid: sugar, caffeine, alcohol, refined carbohydrates, allergens that may cause an allergic reaction, such as peanuts, fish, eggs or milk.

Lifestyle: eat regularly and never rush meals, take regular gentle exercise, avoid stressful situations if possible, use stress management techniques such as meditation and breathing, avoid recreational drugs.

POSTNATAL DEPRESSION; A SOURCE OF SHAME

The mental health issue is so much bigger than Lucy. Her case was very extreme, but postnatal depression is far from uncommon. According to the Joe Bingley Memorial Foundation, 'dedicated to raising awareness and de-stigmatising postnatal depression', in 2009 there were 105,937 new mothers in England and Wales who suffered from postnatal depression, 21,187 of them severely.[2] All of them would have had a terrible time, even though there is a hormone treatment that could help many of them.

A recent very public case was that of the singer Adele. Despite her phenomenal success as a recording artist, she suffered from quite severe depression after her baby was born. In a recent interview with *Vanity Fair* she said: 'You don't want to be with your child; you're worried you might hurt your child; you're worried you weren't doing a good job. But I was obsessed with my child. I felt very inadequate; I felt like I'd made the worst decision of my life.'[3] What a terrible way for a new mother to feel.

Plenty of women can identify with how Adele felt, but their postnatal depression stays hidden out of ignorance, embarrassment, shame or fear of being thought of as a bad mother. The spectrum of symptoms can range from a few days of weepy low mood, through more severe despondency and feelings of inadequacy to a full-blown post-partum psychosis such as Lucy experienced.

There is nothing mysterious about what is going on. It's set out in textbooks and articles. During pregnancy, your progesterone levels can soar to forty times above normal, keeping you calm and happy. Right after birth, they drop to nearly zero, having a knock-on effect on the neurotransmitters and brain chemistry that control moods and emotions.

Cases like Lucy's make clear the urgent need to apply much more widely what we know about the connection between hormones and the brain and emotions. Because it is not something unique to pregnancy. A very similar situation can occur during

---

2   Joe Bingley Memorial Foundation, 'The Incidence of Postnatal Depression'. Available at: http://www.joebingleymemorialfoundation.org.uk/wp-content/uploads/The-Incidence-of-PND-Reports-and-Gaps-in-Services.pdf.
3   https://www.vanityfair.com/culture/2016/10/adele-cover-story

menopause and after a hysterectomy. Once the womb and ovaries are removed, production of both oestrogen and progesterone stops dead. The effects are all too predictable, but official advice on how to treat it can make the situation worse.

The womb isn't just for babies

When my patient Roslyn had to have a total hysterectomy at the age of thirty, she was propelled into early 'surgical' menopause and succumbed to a tidal wave of hormone fluctuations. One day she had her whole complement of hormones – oestrogen, progesterone and testosterone; she woke up after surgery with none, as her ovaries were also removed.

CASE STUDY: ROSLYN

Roslyn was a 46-year-old entrepreneur when she first came to my clinic for help with menopausal symptoms that were having a detrimental impact on her work and family life. Her problems had begun sixteen years earlier, when she had been diagnosed with cervical cancer and had to undergo a complete hysterectomy. Luckily she had given birth to twins three years before the operation. After surgery, she had been put on HRT and tried countless alternative remedies for her symptoms, which included hot flushes, panic attacks, stress and anxiety, but none had made a significant difference. She was despairing of ever finding an effective treatment when she read in a magazine about bio-identical hormones.

Roslyn told me: 'It was a complete shock to go from feeling fit and well to suddenly feeling awful and continuously tired and having hot flushes and panic attacks.' Her GP kept prescribing oestrogen delivered in different ways – patches, implants, tablets and gels – but they either didn't work or would make her feel sick. The hot flushes continued, and she was anxious all the time. She also put on a lot of weight.

'*It was so frustrating and depressing as no one knew anything about it and no one understood what it's like to be in the menopause at thirty. At times I doubted my own sanity and did wonder if it was worth living any more.'*

These feelings were hardly surprising. Trying to pursue a career while looking after two small children and feeling constantly fatigued and unwell must have been an enormous challenge.

When Roslyn's ovaries were removed, she stopped producing her sex hormones – oestrogen, progesterone and testosterone. We saw in Chapter Two how important these hormones are for our brain chemistry. That's why she was constantly anxious. She lacked progesterone, the neurosteroid she needed to stimulate GABA, the main tranquillising neurotransmitter in the brain. She was getting oestrogen from her HRT, but as we've seen earlier, a raised level of oestrogen that isn't balanced by progesterone creates its own set of problems. However, medical wisdom, for some erroneous reason, still dictates that if a woman does not have a uterus, then there is no need for her to be prescribed progesterone.

We've known for twenty years that progesterone must be given with oestrogen in HRT to protect the womb from cancer. It doesn't require much of an imaginative leap to understand that the brain also needs protecting. The leap I find hard to understand is the idea that if a woman has stopped producing three or more hormones, you only need to replace one of them for her to be fine. Every woman undergoing a hysterectomy needs all of them replacing, because it is the right balance of all our hormones that we require to be at our very best.

Roslyn's blood tests revealed excessively high oestrogen levels (from her HRT) but no progesterone or testosterone to balance things. This was a double whammy, as both high oestrogen levels and low progesterone levels can cause anxiety and panic attacks. She needed progesterone for her moods and peace of mind and to balance her oestrogen levels. She also needed it to help her lose weight. She had put on ten kilos since starting on oestrogen therapy and couldn't budge the weight at all.

As well as maintaining mood, rest and sleep, progesterone is also a natural diuretic, and counterbalances the bloating and fluid retention that may be caused by oestrogen dominance. I prescribed Roslyn progesterone and testosterone and recommended that she go on the anxiety protocol (see p.119 above) plus chromium for blood sugar levels and B vitamins for energy. She and others with the same symptoms might also benefit from slightly different diet and lifestyle combinations.

ANXIETY AND LOW ENERGY PROTOCOL

Nutrients: magnesium (essential for muscles, nerve function and sleep), flaxseed oil, also known as hemp oil (high in the plant version of omega-3 fats; some studies finds it reduces inflammation), rhodiola extract, also known as arctic or golden root (used in traditional herbal medicine to improve mood and reduce the effects of stress), L-theanine (an amino acid found in green tea that has a calming effect), chromium picolinate (a trace mineral that helps regulate blood sugar by making insulin more effective, benefiting mood), B vitamins (vital for a healthy nervous system and may help with anxiety and depression).

Eat more: complex carbohydrates, vegetables (especially dark leafy greens), fruits, nuts and seeds, whole grains, oily fish.

Reduce or avoid: sugar, caffeine, alcohol, refined carbs, allergens.

Lifestyle: eat regularly and never rush meals, take regular gentle exercise, avoid stressful situations if possible, use stress management techniques such as meditation and breathing, avoid recreational drugs.

The combination of hormones and lifestyle changes had a dramatic impact on Roslyn's life. She lost weight, she no longer felt depressed or exhausted. Her enthusiasm and positive outlook returned. A year later, she walked the Great Wall of China for charity. She told me: 'There is no way I could even have contemplated something like that before I went on the bio-identical hormones that were compounded specially for me.'

In my opinion, hysterectomies are performed much too readily. For Roslyn it may have been a life-saver, but many women have them for much milder and perfectly treatable problems, such as heavy bleeding. It's a serious operation; patients need around three months' recovery before they are fit to return to work, according to the Hysterectomy Association. It is also surprisingly common – 56,000 in the years 2011 and 2012.[4]

I think there is an attitude that regards the womb as just a place for growing babies. Women are told too often that they no longer need their womb after having had their children. This completely ignores the major role it plays in the female psyche and the importance of the hormones produced by the ovaries in controlling moods and emotions in the brain. It also shows a lack of interest in the way women's physiology works and what they might need medically to function at their best.

---

4   http://www.hysterectomy-association.org.uk/research/latest-hysterectomy-statistics-in-uk-for-the-year-2011-to-2012/

There doesn't seem to be much consideration either of the fact that the whole pelvic region is physiologically one body part. The womb plays an integral part in maintaining stability and proper functioning of the organs in the pelvis. If you remove it, either the rectum or bladder can prolapse, causing a whole new set of medical problems and discomfort for the patient.

For me this suggests a casual disregard for a woman's right to the best possible care, a hangover from the long history of brutal treatment of women with psychological problems that we now understand to very likely have been hormonal. (This subject is covered in Chapter Seven.) In the 1930s, for instance, it was possible for a husband to have his wife committed to an insane asylum for life.

Locked away for life because of her hormones

Vivienne Haigh-Wood Eliot was the wife of the distinguished poet T. S. Eliot. She was certainly a difficult and erratic woman and may well have been, as various reports described her, manipulative, unfaithful, paranoid and maybe even psychotic, but these symptoms were recurring and cyclical over many years and she was plainly suffering from massive hormonal turbulence.

Her mercurial, exaggerated personality may have been initially attractive to Tom Eliot, the impoverished American studying at Oxford, but the allure soon wore off. On their honeymoon, after a brief courtship and secret marriage in 1915, we learn from Vivienne's letters that her period arrived and she flooded the bed sheets with blood. Her new husband spent the night on a deck-chair on Eastbourne beach. She had a habit of changing her bed linen twice a day, and on this occasion even took the sheets home to wash them, causing consternation when the hotel accused her of stealing them.

With the benefit of hindsight, we can see the telltale signs of a hormonal problem. Her symptoms of heavy and irregular periods, being flighty and moody, having fainting spells and migraines are consistent with oestrogen dominance or spiking oestrogen levels and a deficiency of progesterone. Unfortunately, these symptoms were not fully understood at the time and Vivienne's mother eventually took her to a doctor, who diagnosed her with 'hysteria'.

When finally, aged forty, she was found wandering the streets in a confused state, her brother, Maurice, agreed to her committal at a mental institution. Eliot never saw her again but funded her place at the asylum till she died in 1947, sad, isolated, paranoid and delusional. Maurice wrote shortly before his own death that 'She was never a lunatic, I'm sure as the day I was born.'[5]

We can never know whether hormone balancing treatment would have helped Vivienne had it been available, but it could well have been the best treatment for her anxiety, bleeding and 'hysteria'. Her volatile and temperamental behaviour was portrayed as madness because she did not suffer in silence as so many women do. In fact she was screaming out for help.

We may be able to comfort ourselves that we don't have asylums any more where embarrassing or inconvenient relatives can be locked away, but there are many Viviennes alive now showing a similar pattern of behaviour who are first treated with antidepressants, and when those don't work, with antipsychotics – heavy tranquillisers whose side effects include weight gain, diabetes, movement disorders, seizures and suicidal feelings.

---

5   https://www.academia.edu/38993533/Why_Speak_of_Love_Vivienne_Eliot_as_Lavinia_in_The_Cocktail_Party

Taking back control

We've now seen the disastrous impact on emotions and behaviour when hormones are seriously unbalanced, especially when, as with Mrs Eliot, no appropriate hormone treatment is considered. The results were equally grim for Lucy and Roslyn when their levels plummeted to the floor virtually overnight. But these are just extreme versions of what is happening all the time to thousands of women as they slide slowly but inexorably into menopause.

As a medical practitioner, it saddens me to observe all the missed opportunities my patients have endured because their doctors, especially GPs, often use very limited options to diagnose and manage their conditions. The quick-fix approach of prescribing antidepressants may be the easiest for hard-pressed GPs, but in my view, it does not address the root cause of the problem or alleviate symptoms permanently.

Menopause needs a full complement of hormones

Teresa was one of these women who needed help but it took her a long time to find the right sort. She was reluctant to take conventional HRT because of the possible breast cancer risk, and it was only a chance reading of an article by the writer Jeanette Winterson that pointed her in the direction of my clinic. Her story illustrates the many ways menopausal woman can respond to hormonal disruption.

CASE STUDY: TERESA

Migraines, lack of sleep, depression, anxiety and hot flushes had become a way of life for 58-year-old Teresa. She was a self-employed writer and aromatherapy teacher and had been suffering from these menopausal symptoms since her early fifties. They were now starting to severely undermine her well-being and quality of life.

Her migraines were almost constant, and together with the hot flushes and anxiety they were playing havoc with her sleep. 'I was getting about four hours a night,' she told me. 'I felt exhausted much of the time. I was lucky I wasn't in a full-time job, so I could fit my writing and teaching around the symptoms.'

Her GP kept trying to prescribe conventional HRT, which she didn't want. Reading Jeanette Winterson's article confirmed her views: 'I didn't want to substitute my declining hormones with something similar but different. I wanted something that was the same.'

A blood test showed that her levels of oestrogen, progesterone, testosterone and DHEA were all effectively zero, which explained the severity of her symptoms. She was prescribed a combination of the four hormones in a lozenge that dissolved slowly in her mouth. This prescription of bio-identical hormones was uniquely tailored for her needs. 'After three or four days my sleep improved, and the hot flushes, anxiety and depression were better,' she said. 'It was like getting my life back.'

MENOPAUSE PROTOCOL

Nutrients: vitamin E (may be beneficial in anxiety and depression), omega-3 (can improve memory, cross-talk between cells and the working of neurotransmitters; may also relieve depression), omega-6 (used by the body to make prostaglandins that help to make hormones and boost nerve performance), vitamin D3 (the combination of calcium and vitamin D may help reduce symptoms of irritability, anxiety and tearfulness), black cohosh (a natural sedative that helps with chronic anxiety, stress, insomnia or non-restful sleep), dong quai, also known as 'female ginseng' (may have an oestrogen-regulating effect and can relieve hot flushes, palpitations and irritability).

Eat more: complex carbohydrates, vegetables (especially dark leafy greens), fruits, nuts and seeds, whole grains, oily fish.

Reduce or avoid: alcohol, caffeine, sugar and salt, processed foods, trans fats, red meat.

Lifestyle: minimise exposure to environmental toxins, use stress management techniques such as meditation and breathing, take regular exercise.

CONTROL STARTS WITH UNDERSTANDING

Teresa's successful treatment shows why we should never blame ourselves if we are feeling hormonal, be it premenstrual tension, perimenopause or menopause. Being hormonal is nothing to be ashamed of and is not our fault. It is the result of the biological fact that women are designed with a complex and subtle hormonal system that can have powerful and emotionally destabilising effects when the cycles shift. This should not be a cause for puzzled hand-wringing over the fact that women are more likely to show signs of depression than men. Imagine how those figures would change if treatment that actually addressed the cause became widely available.

But we can also alleviate the consequences of our fluctuating hormones if we start asking ourselves why this is happening to us. The answer lies with our brain chemistry, which was discussed in Chapter Two. Once we realise that we are not going mad or just growing old, we can find ways to get our zest and vitality back.

Antidepressants are often only a short-term bandage. We must keep reminding ourselves of the causes of our mood swings. That as well as fluctuating hormones, other factors such as lifestyle and nutrition play a role and are things we can change, as discussed in Chapter Four.

Our monthly hormonal rhythm brings its own changes, but the majority of us deal with it and get on with our lives, our work and our families. However, once you reach the menopause, your hormones are inexorably declining, the symptoms can start to pile up and more specific hormonal help is needed. Among the conditions most likely to trigger a call for help are mood swings and hot flushes, but there are many other disorders that can be greatly helped or even stopped with the correct combination of bio-identical hormones.

Hormonal cocktail can help with migraine

Cindy was menopausal and was getting migraines that were stopping her working for six days a month. She also wanted to avoid HRT because of the cancer risk and because her mother had taken HRT but still suffered from bad symptoms and ended up having a hysterectomy.

CASE STUDY: CINDY

Cindy, a self-employed nurse, had been suffering for the past two years with increasing headaches and migraines and was feeling unusually tired and drained. Her headaches were lasting two days, accompanied by vomiting, and this was happening three or four times a month. She said: 'My GP prescribed anti-epileptic drugs, anti-sickness medication and a drug to narrow the blood vessels in my brain, but nothing worked. The tiredness was extreme. I once closed my eyes at the wheel of the car and mounted the pavement on my way home from work.'

She was also feeling generally unmotivated, with 'brain fog', and could no longer multitask as she used to. She had what she described as 'pain in my bones', with constantly aching neck, hips and lower back. Getting out of bed, the soles of her feet hurt. When she came to see me, she was in a desperate state.

Her blood tests showed she had the same widespread decline in hormone levels that Teresa had suffered. After two weeks of individual replacement therapy, the change was dramatic. She started feeling 'well' again. The cocktail of drugs from her doctor hadn't worked because it was aimed at the wrong target. Hormones were the cause of her malaise and headaches. Later she told me: 'I have so much more energy now and I haven't had a headache or migraine for more than three months.'

Early menopause

Another time when women can have unbalanced and rapidly declining hormones is when the perimenopausal phase comes much earlier than normal. Because it's not expected, even a doctor who is aware of the effect of hormonal changes might miss the real cause of such common symptoms as fatigue, insomnia and anxiety, meaning that confusion and delay in diagnosing it is common. One helpful and informative move your doctor could make would be to do a simple hormone profile. Many women want to know what phase of their life they are at, how their hormones are functioning and how that's making them feel. It's also a very positive step towards a greater understanding of what makes you tick!

CASE STUDY: JULIA

Julia was an ambitious young lawyer who, at thirty-four, was suddenly hit by a blizzard of symptoms but had no idea why. She had never had much time for a personal life and was largely unaware of the rhythm of her periods. Her concern was that the lack of sleep and anxiety were beginning to impact on her work.

Julia came to see me because she did not feel right. She complained of insomnia and had frequent attacks of palpitations, especially at night. In the morning, she was exhausted and couldn't cope with work. She became very teary when she described how anxious she was about her reputation at work and how she had lost confidence in her own abilities. A blood test revealed she was no longer ovulating, so she was no longer producing the combination of oestrogen and progesterone that would normally have kept her functioning harmoniously for another ten or fifteen years.

She didn't know enough to ask her GP to check her hormone levels – even though her symptoms were textbook signs of a deficiency. The chances that a GP would have tested her, however, were small. Instead she would have been offered a range of drugs – antidepres-

sants, sleeping pills, anti-anxiety medication – none of which would have done much good. She might even have been forced to give up her career, all because doctors are still not connecting hormonal imbalance with mental imbalance. Without a bio-identical practitioner she would have faced a grim future.

The early onset of menopause meant that Julia was no longer fertile, something that was very traumatic for her. Grieving the loss of her fertility and what she felt was the loss of her womanhood, she went to see a therapist. With the help of an individualised prescription of hormones and the therapy, she re-established the connection to her female self, and was also able to continue with all the benefits of her own naturally occurring hormones. This was immensely reassuring for her as she wanted to keep her monthly cycle and feel like a 'normal' woman of her age.

Julia's world and her perception changed along with her emotional well-being because of her early menopause. She was no longer ovulating and therefore her ovaries were producing less oestrogen and progesterone. She no longer benefited from the calming effect of progesterone nor from the positive brain-boosting attributes of oestrogen. Hormones have continuous and specific neurological effects on our brains, thus shaping our cognitive and emotional functions at key phases of our life. But what does this mean? Simply put, it means that the interrelationship between our hormones and our mind and mood will not stay the same during our lifetime. They are in an intricate and delicate relationship that we should pay attention to and manage actively. They affect how we feel, how we perceive ourselves, how we relate to our environment and how we respond to the stimuli around us and therefore our very perception of reality. Everything can change when hormones are depleted and no longer exercise their neuroactive responsibilities.

A growing scientific base for the use of bio-identical hormones

The case studies in this book are not exceptions. An analysis of patients treated at the Marion Gluck Clinic shows that around 80 per cent of them have benefited from a prescription of bio-identical hormones. Many no long suffer the symptoms they arrived with. Clinics in America also report a high success rate – one of the factors stimulating the rising popularity of bio-identical hormones. They now make up nearly 50 per cent of hormone replacement prescriptions in the USA.

So there are enlightened doctors who are aware that premenstrual and perimenopausal disruptions are caused by not enough progesterone and changing levels of oestrogen. Sadly, though, this is not yet common knowledge amongst the medical community. The result is that both problems are often falsely ascribed to either lack of oestrogen or an intolerance to progesterone. In such cases oestrogen replacement therapy, oestrogen implants or the oral contraceptive pill can be erroneously prescribed.

This is all wrong, because it doesn't tackle the underlying problem. If there is not enough progesterone to balance the oestrogen, prescribing more oestrogen is likely to make the symptoms worse, while the synthetic form of progesterone (progestins) – found in the oral contraceptive pill and HRT – may even cause increased depression and mood swings, side effects that are listed in the information leaflet inside a packet.

Some American physicians are researching this more sophisticated level of understanding. One of these is Dr Phyllis Bronson, PhD, biochemist and clinician and adjunct associate professor at the University of Denver. She has written that 'high levels of oestrogen produce an imbalance in the system that aggravates or causes symptoms of tension and anxiety'. She agrees that some women with high oestrogen levels may be predisposed to anxiety and even panic attacks.[6] On the other hand, low levels of oestrogen can lead to episodes of depression too. Oestrogen is a 'Goldilocks' hormone – for the best effects, the amounts must be just right – which is why fluctuations can cause such havoc.

Dr Elizabeth Lee Vliet, founder of Hormone Health Strategies in Tucson, Arizona, reported on research carried out at The Rockefeller University that steroid hormones, especially oestrogen, testosterone and progesterone, are the most potent chemical signals affecting the brain. Changes in the levels of these ovarian hormones influence neurotransmitters such as dopamine and serotonin and can have a negative effect on mood and cognitive function.[7]

There's now good evidence that oestrogen is protective against decline in mental function as it 'promotes brain cell survival, growth and regeneration'. Research also suggests that oestrogen could be considered a 'protector against age-related brain decline'.[8]

There is obviously an urgent need to start implementing this growing understanding.

---

6   Phyllis J. Bronson, PhD; 'Mood Biochemistry of Women at Mid-Life' presented at the American Academy of Environmental Medicine Conference, September 28–October 1, 2000.
7   Elizabeth Lee Vliet, MD; 'New insights on hormones and mood', *Menopause Management,* June/July 1993.
8   Claudia Barth, et al., 'Sex hormones affect neurotransmitters and shape the adult female brain during hormonal transition periods', *Frontiers in Neuroscience,* 20 February 2015. Available at: https://doi.org/10.3389/fnins.2015.00037.

Havoc caused by hormonal disrupters

A better-informed account of what causes hormonal problems and how best to treat them is also needed because of the complicated interplay between our hormones and so-called 'hormonal disrupters' found in the environment. These are compounds that can have a direct effect on our hormones, including the tens of thousands of chemicals created and released into the environment over the last seventy years. Some, such as BPA (bisphenol A, see p.187), mimic oestrogen and can disrupt the way the hormone acts in the body. BPA has been associated with higher levels of anxiety, depression, hyperactivity and aggression in children (see p.187). Yet its effects are largely ignored by clinicians. We live in a world where these disrupters are on the rise. Other disrupters include our diet, chemicals in the water, changes in our genes and lifestyle, and especially stress, which can also cause a dip in levels of both our hormones and the feel-good neurotransmitter serotonin.

Becoming empowered

When we ask for help for hormonal symptoms, how often have we been told to 'just get on and deal with it'? But the good news is that we can do something about it. We can become empowered.

Just as we took control of our sexuality and fertility in the 1960s, our greater knowledge today of the way hormones work creates the possibility for taking back control of them. By knowing ourselves and our bodies we can understand our moods, emotions and behaviours better and protect ourselves from the impact of the hormonal ride. As we understand what a key role our hormones play in how we feel, it makes sense to see a doctor who understands the subject and who will help to treat any imbalances with bio-identical hormones. It is very satisfying for me to be able to help women back to where they could and should be in their physical and mental well-being. I just wish more GPs offered this option to their patients.

Meanwhile, you can become aware of the disrupters and take steps to reduce them in your life; you can also track your hormonal changes, learn to handle stress better and eat a hormone-friendly diet. I do hope that this encourages you and makes sense to you. You will find out how I advise you to do all this in Chapter Nine.

SUMMARY OF KEY POINTS

- Statistics show women are more vulnerable to depression than men.
- Should we demand hormonal support or does that play to the stereotype of women as weaker?
- Case study: childbirth and a serious hormone crash triggers a suicide bid with baby.
- Anxiety protocol: food and lifestyle changes can help with anxiety.
- Postnatal depression is a big problem if not properly treated.
- Wombs are not just for babies. Hysterectomies should be a last resort.

- Anxiety and low energy protocol: food and lifestyle changes can help.
- Case study: locked away for life because of her hormones.
- Menopause protocol: food and lifestyle changes can help with symptoms of the menopause.
- Successful treatment of hormonal imbalance needs to deal with the underlying cause. Antidepressants are a short-term solution.
- Bio-identical hormone supplementation can help with menopausal migraine.
- Early menopause is hard to diagnose.
- 80 per cent of patients at the Gluck Clinic have had a positive response to bio-identical hormone therapy.
- We are surrounded by new-to-nature chemicals that can mimic and disrupt our hormones.

CHAPTER SIX

BEYOND PMS AND MENOPAUSE

● ● ● ●

Women have been empowered to take control of their fertility and sexuality in the past. Today, the knowledge is available for women to manage their hormones and have a better quality of life. Of course this is quite a task, because our environment and stressors also play a major role in the way we feel and behave, and these affect our hormones too.

So far we have mostly concentrated on the main sex or reproductive hormones – oestrogen and progesterone – and the effect they can have on moods and emotions in the brain when they become unbalanced. But there are several other hormones that have only been briefly mentioned that can also affect our emotional state and help with various health problems. In this chapter, I'm going to be covering testosterone, cortisol, DHEA and the thyroid hormones T4 (thyroxine) and T3 (liothyronine).

Testosterone and moods

Did you know that men and women have exactly the same hormones flowing through their bodies and affecting their physical and mental functions? The only difference is that we have them in different amounts. Oestrogen is the primary hormone for women and testosterone for men.

Both sexes are surprised when I explain that men at the age of sixty naturally have much more oestrogen than women of the same age. The simple explanation is that as men age, their testosterone is converted into oestrogen. That may be why they are less afflicted with Alzheimer's disease than women, as their brains are protected by oestrogen for longer.

Some experts say women should take oestrogen and progesterone to protect their brains. I think it's a great idea. Research also suggests that testosterone may have a beneficial effect on memory, so let's add that to the mix.

You may be interested to see how similar the chemical structures of oestrogen and testosterone are, even though they have such different effects on different parts of the body and brain. Testosterone is a direct precursor of oestradiol. The two molecules differ from each other by one hydrogen molecule only.

Let's see if you can spot the difference.

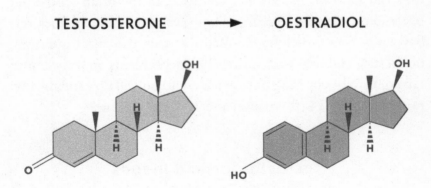

The conversion of testosterone to oestrogen is initiated by an enzyme called aromatase. Aromatase can have an unwelcome effect on men as they get older and their testosterone production starts dropping. The enzyme speeds up the decline, and the extra oestrogen leads to more fat being laid down round the middle. Then, as if that wasn't bad enough, that fat begins to pump out an enzyme that also turns testosterone into fat. And so the waistline spreads and the risk of diabetes and heart problems rises.

The importance of testosterone in men

The drop in testosterone with age can make men bad-tempered and negative. Doctors are generally reluctant to prescribe any replacement, but my experience is that it can be very beneficial.

CASE STUDY: JACK

Jack was a 45-year-old manager and a workaholic. He was driven by success, which was what defined him. He was a family man but admitted that he could have been a better husband and father. He was absent from many of the important family milestones. He missed school events and social occasions and often did not stay on holidays for the allotted time due to work commitments.

Recently he had started having problems at work. He had become increasingly short-tempered with his team, having fits of anger even in front of his clients, and he could not meet the objectives that were set for him. His performance faltered, as did his zeal for the work he was doing. He lacked concentration and energy and no longer felt like his former self. He felt like a failure and started questioning himself as a man, a father and a professional.

He went to see his GP because he thought he might be depressed and need some sort of help. Luckily he had a very open-minded GP, who recognised these symptoms and suggested he test his hormone levels. Jack came to see me, and much to his surprise, his blood tests confirmed his testosterone was low, which was contributing to his behaviour at home and work and explained his declining self-confidence.

Within four weeks of starting testosterone therapy, his self-confidence returned and his mental state improved. Jack is an example of how our mental and physical states are intertwined.

I've had quite a few men in my clinic who have been initially reluctant to admit they need help or discuss symptoms. It's usually their partners who have sent them. Men lose their confidence and their libido in the same way women do, but perhaps a little bit later. There are just as many clichés and jokes about men as they age as there are about women, but now we all know that our emotions are not a joking matter and need to be treated seriously.

For years experts have warned that supplementing with testosterone could either trigger prostate cancer or encourage an established cancer there to grow. Recent research suggests this is unlikely to be a risk.[1]

Women and testosterone

We have seen how the testosterone/oestrogen imbalance can affect men, so how does it affect women? What do we need testosterone for? Should we fear it or embrace it?

---

1 American Urological Association, 'Meta-analysis: Testosterone Is Not a Risk for Prostate Cancer, But . . ', Annual Meeting, 2015.

I often tell my patients that testosterone is a vital female hormone affecting our confidence, mood, self-esteem, motivation, energy, strength, endurance, ability to focus, bone density, libido and sexual function. So it is crucial for us to maintain the balance between oestrogen, progesterone and testosterone as we age and our hormone levels begin to decline.

One of the most common symptoms that women of all ages complain about in my clinic is low libido and lack of confidence. That certainly surprised me in the early days of my practice, but no longer.

How is it possible that low sex drive is so common? A clue is that this is usually not the only symptom. Patients are often also fatigued, and have low energy and little motivation. They don't come across as vital, enthusiastic and confident personalities. In fact, they appear melancholic or slightly anxious and insecure. If the pattern had not become so familiar, I would have said they were depressed.

Something else is going on. As well as lacking the testosterone linked with their sex drive, they often also have low levels of the related androgen hormone DHEA. Their symptoms are commonly mistaken for signs of an underlying depression, because low levels of DHEA bring down mood, energy and sexual desire. Unfortunately, if they receive antidepressants to treat their mood, this can often create a vicious circle, because one of the side effects of antidepressants is low libido.

Today we know that many premenopausal and postmenopausal women suffer from androgen deficiency. In the past, decreased libido was often put down to stress and depression, and instead of being offered blood tests to examine androgen levels, many women were misdiagnosed and did not receive the treatment they needed.

CASE STUDY: CELIA

Celia came to my clinic after having seen her GP and various other therapists to help her with her low libido. She was thirty-eight years old and had been in a relationship for eighteen months. Both she and her partner desperately wanted to have children. Although she adored Joseph, she was very upset that she didn't experience the same sexual desire as she had done in her previous relationships and couldn't understand why. She thought it might be because she was stressed at work and busy organising their wedding, so she decided to see a psychologist. Her GP had already diagnosed her with stress and depression and wanted to prescribe antidepressants. Fortunately, after a few sessions of psychotherapy, her psychologist recommended that she have a blood test for her hormones and thyroid function.

I took Celia's medical and menstrual history. Her periods were always regular, and she didn't suffer any PMS symptoms. In fact, they only lasted two days and she never noticed when they were coming. As they were regular, I could do her blood tests on day twenty-one of her cycle. This is the luteal phase of the cycle, and is the time of the month when we can best identify how efficiently the ovaries are performing and whether they are producing the right amounts of hormones.

Celia's blood tests for oestrogen and progesterone were normal. However, the level of the two androgen hormones (made in her adrenal glands) – testosterone and DHEA – were very low. DHEA isn't as well known as testosterone. It's a life-affirming hormone that gives drive and a zest for life. We make a lot when we are young, but production drops off as we get older. As well as being made in the

144

adrenal glands, testosterone also comes from the ovaries, and can be made from DHEA in peripheral fat tissues.

Celia's lack of testosterone, given her symptoms, was not a surprise. I prescribed DHEA and testosterone cream, as she was severely deficient in both, which was not normal for her age. She received a 25mg DHEA capsule to be taken in the mornings and a testosterone cream that I asked her to apply to her vulva and clitoris once a day after taking a shower.

When Celia walked into my room for her follow-up appointment, she was smiling and appeared more confident. She said that she felt as if her spark had returned. She was still working hard but didn't feel drained at the end of the day and had a twinkle in her eye. She confided that she had had some very lustful nights with Joseph and had started catching herself daydreaming about sex and looking forward to more.

Testosterone was critical for Celia's well-being and mental health. She needed it to stimulate her brain's sex centre, the amygdala, to initiate sexual interest and arousal. She wanted to feel sexy but didn't have the adequate hormonal resources to experience those feelings. With testosterone supplementation, her confidence returned and she was at peace with herself physically and mentally. She learnt to 'let go' a little bit.

Many women don't realise how important testosterone is for our libido. I enjoy watching the reaction of some of my friends and patients when I tell them it is a female hormone. In fact, quantitatively, women produce more androgens than oestrogens. Who would have guessed that? During puberty, girls produce more testosterone than oestrogen.

The importance of testosterone in women is sadly overlooked and underrated. Complaints about lack of sexual interest, difficulty in achieving orgasm and even an aversion to physical or sexual touch is not uncommon. Libido in women starts to decline in their thirties, as does their testosterone production. This is what happened to Celia.

Testosterone replacement therapy is not available in the UK. It was taken off the market in the USA in 2013, even though its beneficial effects have been proven and it can significantly improve a woman's quality of life. It seems a very unsatisfactory state of affairs when men can be prescribed Viagra with ease, but women can have no help if they suffer from low libido.

One of my patients recently said to me, 'Hormonal balance is important so that we can be the person we want to be and know we can be.' I thought this was very true and so succinct. Hormones are hugely important in our lives, always in concert with one another, and only sometimes in isolation. Women and men all have the same complement of steroid sex hormones; the difference lies in the levels that suit our persona and physiology best.

Testosterone and diet and lifestyle

As well as supplementing with testosterone, you can also improve your levels by paying attention to your diet. Make sure you eat ample amounts of healthy carbohydrates such as brown rice, oatmeal, wholewheat bread and pasta, ancient grains such as oats and spelt and sweet potatoes. You also need to include saturated fats such as butter and coconut oil, unsaturated fats – olive oil and omega-3 – and cholesterol.

Don't worry about heart disease: the cholesterol that comes from foods such as eggs, liver, bacon and cheese doesn't affect levels in your blood. Remember that cholesterol is the basic building block of all your sex hormones, including testosterone.

You need plenty of protein from the likes of fish or organic milk, or if you're vegetarian, go for black beans, wild and brown rice, and high-protein fruits and vegetables such as avocados, goji berries, hemp and chia seeds.

Ashwagandha is an Indian herb said to raise testosterone and lower the stress hormone cortisol, as well as improving the immune response and helping with insomnia and fatigue.

Finally, if you are focusing on increasing your testosterone go easy on flax or hemp seeds (unless you're vegetarian, in which case, you'll need the added fibre these seeds bring). Recommended for their high levels of fibre and some minerals, they also contain lots of lignan, a plant compound that pushes up oestrogen and brings down testosterone. For women with an excess of testosterone, however, they could be the answer.

DHEA, the *joie de vivre* hormone for mood and energy

DHEA has many nicknames: the longevity hormone, the super hormone, the fountain of youth hormone and the mother of all hormones. I call it the *joie de vivre* hormone, as in my medical experience, people with high levels of DHEA are more positive, enthusiastic and have a zest for life. I prescribe it very frequently in my practice for both women and men for the same reasons: energy and well-being. DHEA is one of the most abundant steroid hormones in both sexes, and is produced in the ovaries, testes and the brain as well as in the adrenal glands. Its main role in the body is as a precursor molecule for the production of oestrogen and androgen, the female and male sex steroid hormones.

It is known that DHEA production peaks at around the age of twenty-five and begins to decline slowly thereafter. This is one of the reasons it is considered by some as an anti-ageing treatment.

We saw earlier how progesterone acts as a neurosteroid in the brain. Well so does DHEA, as it binds to receptor sites. Research published in the journal *Nature* in 2013 found that DHEA improved the connections between the amygdala, where emotional responses are controlled, and the hippocampus, essential for memory, and calmed down brain cell activity in both regions.[2] These changes are thought to be associated with both improvement in mood and a reduced memory for negative emotional events. It may have an effect in lifting depression.

Another reason why DHEA may be considered anti-ageing is that it is involved in protecting nerve cells from toxins and injury that may occur, for example, after a stroke. At the moment, a great deal of research on DHEA is taking place. In theory, DHEA could slow down the ageing process, improve well-being, cognitive function and body composition and may be effective in treating depression.

So if we are feeling run down or sad, or we're not coping with daily events, it's not necessarily that something is wrong with us; it may very well be that something is wrong with our hormones. Either we don't have enough of them, or they are not in balance and are fluctuating and unstable.

DHEA is claimed to improve physical performance, and although more research needs to take place, it is a banned substance amongst athletes because it is considered to be an anabolic steroid. In the USA, it is available over the counter as a supple-

---

2   Rebecca K Sripada et al., 'DHEA Enhances Emotion Regulation Neurocircuits and Modulates Memory for Emotional Stimuli', *Neuropsychopharmacology*, 2013, Vol. 38, pp.1798–1807.

ment in pharmacies and supermarkets. Considering it is a powerful hormone, one wonders about the wisdom in classing DHEA as such, whilst at the same time the World Anti-Doping Agency classes it as a banned substance. It is, after all, a hormone and needs to be treated with understanding and respect.

CASE STUDY: STEVEN

Steven was in his late forties and was sent to me by his partner, Ella, who was complaining that he had become a grumpy old man and was no longer fun to be with. Ella was also a patient of mine and booked him in because she thought he might be suffering from depression but didn't want to face the fact.

Steven explained that he had been feeling low for the last eighteen months. He had lost interest in his work and was underperforming not only at work but also at home. He was less attentive with Ella and his libido was low. He told me that he could quickly become very irritable and a sense of anger was never far off. He no longer enjoyed socialising or travelling and had also stopped exercising. He slept badly and felt constantly fatigued. He realised that he was feeling depressed but acknowledged that there was no reason for this.

Ella wanted her husband back and I was pretty sure that if we checked his hormones and thyroid function, we would find the reason for his woes. Sure enough, his blood test results showed that his testosterone was low, though still in the normal range. Normal only tells you what most people have. There is no guarantee that it is right for any one person, especially if they have the symptoms linked with low levels. Steven's DHEA was also very low, certainly lower than expected at his age. I prescribed him 100mg of DHEA. I generally expect testosterone to improve when I prescribe DHEA in sufficient amounts because the body can and does make testosterone from it. (This happens in both men and women, and we are genetically programmed to produce the amount our gender requires.)

When I reviewed Steven six weeks later, his whole demeanour was different. He walked into my room smiling and looking confident and said that he couldn't believe how different he felt. He was at peace with himself, and no longer irritable. He was sleeping better and had regained an enthusiasm for his work.

When Steven returned for his three-month review, he told me that he was back to being the manager he had been before. He happily commented that his sex life had also improved, he had lost his paunch and had started running again. Steven and Ella continue to be my patients. After a year, I added testosterone into Steven's prescription because he felt he wanted more physical energy and mental focus for work. With DHEA, his zest for life had returned and his mood and motivation had improved, and with the addition of testosterone, his drive, energy and mental acuity returned. He felt great and content with his life.

DHEA is just as important for women as it is for men. Ella also had DHEA in her prescription to give her the joie de vivre she wanted.

Steven might well have benefited from a nutrition and lifestyle combination designed to provide support for the adrenal hormones – his testosterone was on the low side and he was deficient in DHEA.

ADRENAL SUPPORT PROTOCOL

Nutrients: Siberian ginseng (increases tolerance of stress and can help in the production and regulation of stress hormones in the adrenal gland), rhodiola extract, also known as arctic or golden root (used in traditional medicine to improve mood and reduce the effect of stress), magnesium (essential for muscles, nerve function and sleep), vitamin C (recent research found it helps reduce the physical and psychological effects of stress and improves the rate of recovery), zinc (important for immunity, wound healing and is needed to produce testosterone) and L-tyrosine (a precursor for the mood-boosting neurotransmitters such as dopamine and is needed to produce thyroid hormones).

Eat more: complex carbohydrates, vegetables, fruits, nuts and seeds, whole grains, oily fish.

Reduce or avoid: sugar, caffeine, alcohol, refined carbohydrates, salt, saturated and trans fats.

Lifestyle: Regular gentle exercise, minimise stress, minimise exposure to environmental toxins, avoid recreational drugs.

A couple of other ideas worth considering are spending time in the sun, because the same process that makes vitamin D (using a form of cholesterol in the skin) also produces DHEA. And avoid having high levels of insulin (suggesting a problem with controlling your blood sugar), because that will reduce the effectiveness of DHEA.

Pregnenolone is another related hormone that is made in the adrenal glands. It has a number of beneficial effects, including enhancing memory and reducing stress-induced fatigue. Pregnenolone is the first stage in making the steroid hormones from cholesterol, mostly in the adrenal glands but also in the brain. It can then be used to make all the other hormones – DHEA, progesterone, testosterone, oestrogens and cortisol – which is why it is sometimes called the mother hormone. It may reduce feelings of being stressed and help you to handle stress better. The result can be improved mood and energy, and less severe symptoms of PMS and menopause. Signs that you are getting too stressed include low body temperature, feeling weak, becoming more irritable, finding it hard to concentrate, being hungry all the time and not sleeping well.

Like DHEA, you make high levels of pregnenolone when you are young, but these decline as you get older, until by sixty-five you are producing only 60 per cent of what you were making at thirty-five. As well as reducing your stress protection, this can lower the levels of all the other hormones that are made from pregnenolone.

Things that will help to keep your levels up include getting enough sleep and regular exercise, as well as eating the sort of healthy diet covered earlier. If you still need help, you can take it in pill form, which may help with those stress symptoms.

What are my hormones up to?

I have a lot of patients who come to me and want to know what their hormone levels are. They may be near the menopause or have always been on the pill and have no idea of their monthly cycle. Some just don't feel like themselves; they know something is changing but don't understand what it is. They would like to know if replacing their hormones is an option, and if so, what they should do about it.

CASE STUDY: VICKY

Vicky was one of these patients. She was a 44-year-old teacher who had been hearing a lot about hormones from her friends. She'd never really bothered to think about them as she had been on the pill most of her life. She was a single mother of a teenage daughter. She'd separated from her husband when her daughter was eight, but the relationship remained amicable and her ex-husband was a responsible and attentive father.

After the separation, she never stopped taking the pill even though she was not in a relationship. She knew she would have to come off it soon and was quite anxious about this as she didn't know what to expect. She came to see me to find out what her hormones were doing and for advice on the menopause. Except for the short period of about two years when she became pregnant, Vicky had never been off synthetic hormones.

There are many women like this who have hardly ever experienced the natural rhythm of their body. Unfortunately, many then find they don't trust their body because of their dependence on the pill. At least the pill is predictable and controlling, and if you tolerate it, then why stop? This is the mindset of many women, but they do not understand that they may be harming their health long term; a risk that is spelt out if you read about the pill's side effects.

I explained to Vicky that the pill would always mask what was going on with her hormones. I advised her to take a break and experience what was happening naturally to her body. I suggested she come back once she'd done that to check her hormones. She agreed, somewhat reluctantly, afraid that she might become as moody as she had been before going on the pill.

After six weeks, she returned, surprised that she felt fine except for some tiredness. In fact, she had even lost a bit of weight, which pleased her as she was beginning to find it difficult to shift any excess pounds. I took her bloods and all her results appeared normal. As she was not in a relationship, I advised her to stay off the pill and start to become acquainted with her body and see how her moods and emotions developed when she was no longer under the influence of an oral contraceptive. She was relieved to find that all was well and was now more confident about staying off it.

I don't try to convince my patients to stop taking the pill, but I explain to them the pros and cons of it. We know that synthetic hormones can have many negative side effects, such as low libido, weight gain and even depression. So why take it if you don't need a contraceptive? Why suppress your natural cycle and miss out on all the beneficial effects of your own hormones if you don't need to?

Vicky returned about eighteen months later. She was having a lot of stress with her teenage daughter and she felt as if she wasn't coping as well as she could. Her periods were regular and short, lasting just two days, and she had very few PMS symptoms. But her moods were up and down, and she was frequently fatigued. Could this have something to do with her hormones? She was feeling easily overwhelmed and had lost enthusiasm for teaching.

This time there was a change in her hormone levels. She was now forty-six and perimenopausal, but it wasn't progesterone or oestrogen that she was lacking; it was DHEA, her adrenal gland hormone. I supplemented this with 15mg daily and she seemed to get her zest back as before and managed her daily stress much better.

Vicky only needed a bit of supplementation to get her balance back. She was pleased that she didn't need to rely on the pill to get a regular cycle. She was also much more confident and knowledgeable about the menopause and what to expect, and had trust in her body to deal with it. This was a situation where a woman decided to take control of her cycle and manage her moods and hormones as required.

Not everyone is as fortunate as Vicky, who was very proactive about getting to know how her body functioned and what to expect from her hormones.

Many women tend to neglect their own needs and prioritise the demands and expectations of the environment around them. Women are mothers, wives, daughters, professionals and workers. Many fulfil all these roles and have the responsibility of satisfying multiple demands at once. We are brilliant at multi-tasking. This is not a cliché; we know it, and studies of the brain have proven it.

But let's face it, it can become exhausting. How do we find the time for ourselves and our own needs? When demands on us become overwhelming, we need to know ourselves and comprehend what resources we have. We have already established that women are most vulnerable at times of hormonal change and fluctuations. The unfortunate thing is that women are seventeen times more likely to be diagnosed with depression in the perimenopause than at any other time of their life. This is of course not a coincidence.

From my experience, the perimenopause, which can last anything from two to eight years, is the most challenging time for both patient and doctor. Managing and balancing hormones is always a work in progress. There are occasions when it all goes wrong at once, and I have had to find a way to help using both conventional and complementary treatments.

Sleep and how a hormone check can help

Many of my patients report problems with sleeping, and one of the issues is often that they are not handling stress very well, which means that hormones are probably involved. Specifically, human growth hormone (HGH) and the stress hormone cortisol.

Patrick Holford, the UK's leading nutrition expert, explains what is going on: 'Sleep provides essential "nourishment" for both body and mind. During the night, and especially during the deep and REM sleep phases, your brain produces higher levels of HGH which helps with the repair that routinely goes on at night.'[3]

When you're stressed, the level of the stress hormone cortisol goes up. You feel agitated and that makes it harder to sleep. The cortisol also suppresses HGH because as far as the body is concerned dealing with the stress has a higher priority. So, energy is diverted away from repair into coping with the stressful situation.

Regularly cutting back on this night-time repair can speed up the ageing process, and that sets up a vicious circle. Slowing down repair is itself stressful, causing more release of cortisol, which keeps the insomnia going.

And it gets worse. Frequent insomnia can make people feel very anxious and depressed, and this too has knock-on effects. If we are feeling depressed, we won't produce enough of the feel-good neurotransmitter serotonin, which is needed to produce our main sleep hormone, melatonin. Another vicious circle. We need to break the cycle of stress and its effect on our neurotransmitters and brain chemistry if we are going to enjoy a healthy night's sleep again.

---

3   https://www.patrickholford.com/advice/power-of-sleep

Fatigue doesn't only cause low mood, it may also make us irritable or short-tempered, and we begin to feel, probably unreasonably, that we can't cope with our daily routines. When I met Agnes, she had got caught up in this negative feedback loop.

CASE STUDY: AGNES

Agnes was a very successful professional woman in her mid forties whose main concern was her sleep. For the last year her sleep pattern had dramatically altered. Every night she went to bed exhausted but then would wake up after about two hours and toss and turn for what seemed like hours. She was beginning to dread going to bed.

She came to me in the hope that her hormones might have something to do with it because then there might be a treatment to try. But she had no idea what her hormones might be doing because she had had a coil called Mirena inserted and hadn't had a period for three years. She even thought she might be menopausal because she had heard that insomnia was a symptom of menopause.

I took blood tests and checked her hormone levels. Her ovaries were still producing the expected amount of oestrogen for her age, but she wasn't producing any progesterone. This meant that she wasn't ovulating. Having low progesterone levels can result in many symptoms. Agnes was fine except for her insomnia, which was affecting her quality of life and work. It was also making her feel anxious and very fatigued. She was of course also perimenopausal, and progesterone is the first hormone that begins to decline as we approach menopause.

I prescribed progesterone cream to be applied transdermally every evening before going to bed. Progesterone in our system breaks down into allopregnanolone, which helps the GABA receptors in the brain to initiate its calming effect and bring about sleep.

She could also have tried my sleep protocol, outlined below, which involves dietary and lifestyle changes that can help.

SLEEP PROTOCOL

Nutrients: B complex (B vitamins are vital for a healthy nervous system and may help with anxiety and depression), magnesium (essential for muscles, nerve function and sleep), calcium (essential for nerve function; levels are higher during deep sleep, and low levels are linked with insomnia), L-theanine (an amino acid found in green tea that has a calming effect), 5-HTP (the raw material for making the neurotransmitter serotonin and also the sleep hormone melatonin). Natural sources of melatonin can be found in bananas, oats, walnuts, liquorice and grape skins and in the herbs sage, fever-few and St John's wort.

Eat more: complex carbohydrates, vegetables (especially dark leafy greens), fruit, nuts and seeds, whole grains.

Reduce or avoid: sugar, caffeine, alcohol, refined carbs.

Lifestyle: take regular gentle exercise, minimise stress, practise relaxation techniques as part of bedtime routine, promote balanced blood sugar as low sugar levels can trigger early waking.

When just hormones are not enough

I hope it is clear by now that replacing declining hormones with bio-identical supplements can be an effective treatment for a wide range of conditions. We've seen how people who have been trying to find help for depression or anxiety for years have experienced major improvements within a few weeks of starting on a BHRT course. But it is not a panacea. Even if you have been prescribed a course you have to remember to take it, and often it will work much better if you combine it with various lifestyle changes that you have to commit to as well.

In addition, you can become distressed or depressed for reasons that have nothing to do with hormonal changes. Some social and psychological factors will never respond to a compounded prescription. Then other resources have to be brought in – the family, a therapist, change of job or environment. There are a few people who react badly to hormone replacements. Not everybody benefits from every treatment and some people have conditions that are just too complicated or challenging for an easy solution. Georgina was one of those people.

CASE STUDY: GEORGINA

When I first saw Georgina, she was 48 and definitely in the peri-menopause. She had just sold her successful fashion label and was exhausted. Her primary complaint was insomnia and feeling stressed, and she wanted to know if taking hormones would help her relax and sleep again.

I took a blood test and her hormones were all over the place. Oestrogen was excessively high, progesterone was zero and testosterone and DHEA were very low.

At the follow-up consultation, she seemed even more anxious and agitated and was demanding a quick fix. After years of hard work, she was now financially independent and wanted to enjoy life. She said her insomnia was driving her crazy.

I explained to her that her symptoms were most likely to be a result of her fluctuating and deficient hormones. She needed progesterone to help her sleep and calm her down and DHEA to give her some energy and motivation.

Georgina, like many women, had been neglecting her own needs, but she was impatient for results and expected a quick fix. She was busy co-parenting her child with her ex-husband; her career, her son and her ageing mother were her priorities now. She found no time to go to counselling or mindfulness classes or yoga, or just to find a peaceful corner for herself. She was also becoming more and more anxious, which she attributed to lack of sleep, even though her GP had reluctantly prescribed sleeping tablets.

I prescribed her DHEA for energy and progesterone to help her sleep. As previously mentioned, studies have shown that progesterone has an anti-anxiety effect by acting on the GABA receptors in the brain.

Unfortunately, Georgina returned two months later, accompanied by her mother, who was genuinely very worried about her. She had become more anxious, irritable and frantic. She was desperate to sleep but the sleeping tablets were no longer working. She wasn't coping at all. She took the hormones and supplements I prescribed irregularly. Because of her anxiety and depressive mood, I had also prescribed the supplement 5-HTP to help improve serotonin levels and magnesium glycinate to calm her down, but she couldn't remember if she had taken them or not.

In the meantime, she had asked her ex-husband to look after her son full time as she wasn't coping at home and was either in tears or irritable and shouting. I recommended that Georgina seek psychiatric help, but to my relief she had already done this and had made an appointment to see a psychiatrist. I also tried to impress upon her the importance of taking the progesterone daily. Unfortunately, she was non-compliant.

I found out that most of Georgina's symptoms were happening in the second week of her cycle. In fact, she felt a bit better only during her periods and for a week after. This narrow window suggested she was suffering from premenstrual dysphoric disorder (PMDD). This is a psychiatric diagnosis in which women suffer from recurrent severe symptoms of depression, tension, irritability and insomnia before their periods. However, in her case it had escalated into a severe perimenopausal depression. She was no longer coping with her anxiety and lack of sleep. She was exhausted and this compounded her depression. Her high oestrogen levels didn't help because we know that oestrogen dominance can cause feelings of anxiety and excitability.

Progesterone therapy is one of the key elements in the treatment of premenstrual tension, PMDD and perimenopausal depression. Progesterone affects the GABA receptors in the brain, which work as an inhibitory neurotransmitter, reducing excitation most likely caused by spiking oestrogen levels. Progesterone promotes GABA activity to induce sleep and relaxation. Poor GABA activity has been linked to low mood, anxiety and sleep disorders. A decrease in GABA results in an increased excitability of the nervous system.

Of course, antidepressants may also play a valuable and key role in treatment of depressive symptoms. Selective serotonin reuptake inhibitors (SSRIs) are the most commonly used. They increase the amount of serotonin in the brain by blocking its reabsorption. SSRIs do not make more serotonin, but they make it more available. This is the reason why I prescribe 5-HTP, as it is a neurotransmitter and direct precursor to serotonin, the feel-good hormone in the brain. The more 5-HTP you have in your system, the more serotonin you can produce.

So, progesterone plus GABA would normally keep someone calm and tranquil, while oestrogen helps increase the level of neurotransmitters, such as serotonin and dopamine, which improve mood. But too much dopamine, which is an excitatory neurotransmitter, and not enough serotonin causes nervousness and anxiety. Balance of all neurotransmitters as well as hormones keeps our brain chemistry functioning harmoniously.

Unfortunately, progesterone therapy and the perimenopausal supplement protocol were no longer sufficient for Georgina. She needed psychiatric treatment and antidepressants and was admitted to hospital as an in-patient to help her sleep and wean her off her sleeping medication, She also needed ways to reduce her anxiety and monitor her mood swings while finding the right medication to modify her overwrought emotional state. While she was in hospital, I continued to prescribe progesterone for her, which her psychiatrist had requested.

Fortunately, after six weeks she was released from the hospital on antidepressant medication that suited her well. She also appreciated the fine nuances of her oscillating hormones and now takes progesterone twice daily to maintain that much-needed sense of calm she had begun to experience.

This was a case where lifestyle, stress and hormonal imbalance together precipitated the decline from mood swings to insomnia to depression. Hormone-balancing therapy, particularly with progesterone, became part of the treatment to help Georgina get her life back. The combination of psychotherapy and the appropriate use of antidepressants, together with a new awareness of ways to handle her life stressors and a knowledge of the role hormones play has reassured Georgina that she is once more the person she wants to be and knows she can be.

Thyroid and moods

When I was in medical school and doing my psychiatry module, our professor got up in front of the room, looked at us very seriously and told us that if we ever considered diagnosing anyone with depression or any other mental health issue, we had to check their thyroid function first.

I listened with disbelief. How could a tiny organ in the neck have anything to do with the way we felt and behaved? I was sure he was making a mistake and so I never forgot his comment and how ridiculous we students thought it was.

Of course the psychiatry professor was right and I was wrong. Studies have proved that a lack of thyroid hormones has been linked with cognitive and mood disorders.

Dr Mark Vanderpump, an eminent UK endocrinologist, confirms that: 'A healthy thyroid plays a vital part in brain chemistry, so we should not be surprised that a thyroid disorder can cause unpredictable mood changes.' He goes on to say: 'If you have an underactive thyroid (hypothyroidism) you may feel stressed and overwhelmed and experience depression, tearfulness, and loss of appetite. Overall you may feel a progressive loss of initiative, a dulling of personality and you may encounter memory problems, difficulty in concentration, muddled thinking and a lack of interest or mental alertness.'

Does this sound like you? I am sure that many of us on occasion have felt this way, but hopefully it has been transitory. As doctors we definitely have to consider thyroid function in the majority of our patients. If you do ever feel this way, you should request that your GP do blood tests and check your thyroid function.

The problem is that an underactive thyroid develops slowly.

Often we try to get used to the fact that we are feeling low, putting on weight or are unreasonably tired. Some of us may put it down to ageing and assume that it is something we have to endure. This is wrong. We all have the right to feel the best we can. Neither ageing nor hormone imbalance should reduce our quality of life.

Studies have shown that psychological well-being improves when hormone levels are raised using hormone therapy. Thyroid hormones have a modulating effect on serotonin in the brain and have a positive influence on our brain chemistry.

Since that first psychiatry lecture I have encountered numerous patients who confirmed that the cause of their 'depression' was a lack of thyroid hormones. It's so rewarding when patients who have tried various treatments for their fatigue, mental fog, low moods and low self-esteem return and say, 'It was like flicking a switch and my brain was turned on again' or 'I feel like myself again and have my life back.'

Most patients with low thyroid symptoms respond very well to the standard treatment with the thyroid hormone T4. But about 10 to 15 per cent are told that, although they have many of the symptoms of low thyroid, because blood tests show their hormone levels in the normal range, they don't have a problem. This is a complex and controversial area, but some of these patients benefit greatly from treatment with another thyroid hormone, T3.

The problem is that the physical symptoms of an underfunctioning thyroid, such as weight gain, hair loss or low libido, compound the symptoms of low esteem and contribute to low mood. As you can, see this is another vicious circle that needs to be broken.

CASE STUDY: MIREILLE

Mireille never felt quite right. She went to her GP often, complaining of fatigue, frequent infections, low mood and never having enough energy. Her bloods were checked but everything came back normal. At times she would feel quite desperate and low that she couldn't enjoy life like others around her. Her GP implied that she might suffer from depression and wrote her a prescription for antidepressants. She tried these only for a short time and felt more like a zombie than before, and her energy did not improve.

I repeated her thyroid blood tests, and although she was in the 'normal' range, her result could still have been much better. After all, she did have many symptoms of an under-functioning thyroid.

I prescribed her the lowest dose of thyroid hormones and advised her to go on the thyroid protocol. Her response was instantaneous! She felt immediately better. Just by topping up her thyroid hormones by a small amount, her moods and energy lifted immediately, as did her thyroid blood tests, which are checked every six months.

Besides replacing and balancing hormones, which you can only do with the help of your doctor, here are some things you can try to support your thyroid function. The right foods and supplements will help improve your symptoms.

As well as thyroid dysfunction, we need to address adrenal disorders here too, as a lot of the symptoms can overlap and be common to both. Luckily treatment with supplements and the right food and lifestyle advice can tackle both conditions.

THYROID PROTOCOL

Selenium is important as it helps the inactive T4 thyroid hormone convert into the active T3 thyroid hormone.

Zinc is a trace element that, together with selenium and copper, is required for the synthesis and conversion of thyroid hormones from T4 to T3. Equally, these hormones are essential for the absorption of zinc and low levels can lead to zinc deficiency.

Tyrosine is an amino acid that is essential for the synthesis of thyroid hormones. It is also necessary for the formation of adrenaline and noradrenaline by the adrenal glands. This is one of the reasons why adrenal stress or adrenal fatigue, whichever way you prefer to refer to it, can impact on thyroid function.

Iodine in combination with tyrosine is needed to make thyroid hormones. A lack of iodine in the diet can lead to an under-functioning thyroid gland. Some foods can block the uptake of iodine by the thyroid gland; they come from the brassica family and consist of cabbage, broccoli and Brussels sprouts. Soya beans, pine nuts and millet can also hinder the absorption of iodine.

Essential fatty acids from fish are important for the function of cell membranes in the thyroid.

Vitamin A, vitamin B complex, vitamin C and vitamin E are all essential for the formation of thyroid hormones.

Lifestyle changes, nutritional foods and the intake of supplements are easy wins and can be the stepping stone to your wellness, with improved mood and quality of life.

SUMMARY OF KEY POINTS

- Men's testosterone turns into oestrogen as they get older.
- Testosterone can boost both men and women's libido, drive and confidence.
- Symptoms of low testosterone can appear very similar to depression.
- Case history of a woman with low libido shows that she was helped with a supplement of energising hormone DHEA, which makes testosterone.
- Improving testosterone levels can be done with diet and life-style.
- DHEA provides energy and feelings of well-being. Levels are high in the young and decline with age. There is research to show DHEA may slow ageing.
- Case history shows DHEA restores libido.
- Adrenal support protocol: diet and lifestyle changes can help those with low testosterone and DHEA.
- Case history of woman who took oral contraceptove pill for decades, which is not uncommon, shows the effects this can have on hormone health.
- DHEA can help long-term pill user to manage stress.
- Hormones can help with damaging effects of insomnia.
- Sometimes hormone supplements are not enough. Psychological problems may also need therapy and drugs.
- Thyroid hormones and mood are closely linked.

CHAPTER SEVEN

WOMEN AND MADNESS: BRUTAL BEGINNINGS THAT STILL RESONATE TODAY

● ● ● ●

Since the feminist movement of the 1960s, the socio-economic situation of women has improved dramatically. The oral contraceptive pill and the control it gave women over their fertility and sex drive was very empowering. The new sense of freedom and emancipation, however, has come at a cost. Women are being challenged to cope with multi-tasking lifestyles, resulting in an increase in stress levels, expectations and responsibilities.

We are also becoming aware of the more profound biological cost of denying our natural bodily rhythms. We have won so much, but has the price been to lose sight of our female selves? Perhaps we have deprived ourselves of understanding the implications of our biology in order to fit into a male-centric universe.

I'm optimistic that the changes don't have to be damaging, because we are starting to understand our hormones, and to pay attention to our cycles and respect our natural bodily rhythms again. We are getting to know ourselves and what makes us tick. We are getting in tune again with our nature. Young women are moving away from controlling their hormones with the oral contraceptive pill; today they are using apps to get their timing right.

Thank goodness times have changed. In the nineteenth century, Victorian women were locked away in asylums and treated with terrible surgical procedures that negated their womanhood. In the twentieth century they were subjected to the Freudian belief that past experiences, deeply embedded in their minds, controlled their bodies. Now we are beginning to draw these strands together and realise that our hormones are the connecting thread.

Hormones keep women out of drug trials

Unfortunately there is still a strong cultural stigma around hormones and being 'hormonal'. Women don't like to talk about it, and many suffer in silence. Hormones – their actions and the way they affect us all – are often misunderstood, and to compound this issue, women are also under-represented in medical research. This has raised the risk that they will suffer harmful side effects from drug prescriptions. Between 1997 and 2001, ten prescription drugs were withdrawn from the American market of which eight where found to pose 'greater health risks for women' because of adverse side effects. [1]

How come this wasn't spotted before the drugs were put on the market? The shocking and surprising reason is that they were never specifically tested for their effect on women. Even though the scientists knew that drugs could have different effects on men and women, most of the subjects in the clinical trials were men.

---

1   https://www.gao.gov/new.items/d01286r.pdf

Historically there has been a bias against including female subjects in medical research projects on the grounds that they could mess up the experiment. Women's fluctuating hormone levels and monthly cycles could alter their response to the drugs, confusing the results. Trying to control for this costs money, making women more expensive test subjects. As a result, it was easier and cheaper to just use males and assume that women were effectively small men. Then the same treatment could be given to both women and men, with dosage adjustments being made on the basis of size rather than gender.

There was a good reason for being cautious about including women in drug trials – the risk of birth defects if they were pregnant, thalidomide being the classic example. But simply excluding them was not the answer. It was an example of an all-too-common brutal response to problems raised by women's different physiology instead of a humane and informed solution. Woman are now being increasingly included in trials, but sadly this historic gender bias has been to the detriment of all of us.

Women's fates and the understanding of their biology could have been so different. Women in the past didn't have that opportunity to know themselves, and issues raised by their biology were too often ignored or treated as aberrations.

Had we been more aware of our bodies and psyche and suffered less interference from Church, politicians, pharmaceutical companies and medical men, we may have done better. A quick overview of what Victorian women faced when they developed psychological problems gives you an idea of the challenges in their path. The callous treatments may be a thing of the past, but the attitudes behind them still linger.

Madness in Victorian times

When I read the views of eighteenth- and nineteenth-century physicians – always men – of women with medical and psychological problems, I am horrified at the repressive and seemingly cruel notions they had, just as I am bemused at the belief systems these evolved from.

Women today cannot comprehend what it means to be treated as a possession, or be valued only for our wombs and hidden away in shame when 'women's problems' send us 'mad', although the current attitude to hysterectomies, covered earlier, shows echoes of an older, harsher response that are still with us.

From the eighteenth century onwards, an epidemic of hysteria, a catch-all term for any unidentified nervous or mental disorder, swept through the women of Europe. Hysteria, which the ancient Greeks identified as a 'wandering womb', became a diagnosis often applied to women's mental problems. Prominent respected men of science spent years researching and pronouncing on this mysterious illness, attempting to back up their frequently idiosyncratic theories with observation and data.

In 1794, in post-revolution Paris, Philippe Pinel took over the Salpêtrière asylum, previously a dumping ground for beggars, prostitutes and 'the alienated', as lunatics were termed. He reputedly established the beginnings of a more humane treatment of the inmates, the vast majority of whom were women. At least he liberated them from their chains!

It's the subconscious that's driving women mad

Pinel's successor, Jean-Étienne Esquirol, kept meticulous notes and recorded links between pregnancy, childbirth and post-partum or 'puerperal' madness, from which at least 10 per cent of his intake suffered. The diagnosis was no respecter of class or wealth, with rich women equally susceptible to this affliction – which, as we have seen, is still not treated in an effective or biolog-ically based way even today.

From 1825, Jean-Martin Charcot and his followers continued to develop the asylum's reputation as a centre for the new specialism of psychiatry, and turned the patients into living experiments. He had over four thousand women under his care, and categorised every mental or nervous system disorder, but his prime interest was in women with hysteria.

It was believed that the 'troubled or wandering' womb could send women into exaggerated or uncontrollable emotions that could drive them insane. Interestingly, a young Sigmund Freud attended Charcot's lectures in 1885, and the ideas he heard dis-cussed there underpinned his development of psychoanalysis, which took a different direction and focused on the power of the unconscious mind to affect the physical body.

Before Freud, there was a general consensus amongst nine-teenth-century men of science that women were the weaker sex and that certain kinds of madness particular to women had a bodily basis. What wasn't at all clear was what could trigger them. A new answer was provided by Freud, who challenged the im-portance of the body and identified the unconscious mind as the driver of madness.

Demand to be taken seriously: a sign of madness

My view is that Freud was right about the link between the mind and madness, or at least the diagnosis of madness, but not quite in the way that he thought. Could the infantilising and medicalising of women by consigning to asylums those with unidentified mental and physical problems be connected to the increasingly loud clamour from other women to be taken seriously as poets and writers, to earn their living independently, to legally control their fortunes and to have the right to vote?

In Victorian literature, there is an ever-growing band of troubled women who feature as fallen women, lunatic women, depressed women or mysterious threatening women. Indeed, the great men (and women) of letters often had personal experience of madness in their families.

William Thackeray's wife had broken down after the birth of their daughter, and attempted to drown her baby and commit suicide. Thackeray had her confined to a madhouse. Wilkie Collins and Charles Dickens both visited asylums, and Collins characterised the instability of women in his tale of *The Woman in White*, whilst Dickens's Lady Dedlock epitomised middle-aged depression and despair.

The coincidence is not lost on me. The more uppity women became in society, the more forcefully their weaknesses were emphasised and the more repressive their treatments seem to have become.

Reading books or playing music can damage a woman's mind

The Victorians were obsessed with 'the woman question'. In both Britain and America renowned physicians were busy investigating the causes of neurasthenia (a kind of lassitude and exhaustion) and hysteria and coming up with more and more extraordinary methods of treating them. According to the famous Victorian doctor Sir Henry Maudsley, too much excitement or exertion was dangerous to women – and that included playing music or reading serious books – the cure was total rest. Sir Henry also wrote in 1874 that women were intellectually handicapped on the grounds that they spent one week of the month 'more or less sick and unfit for hard work'. [2]

We no longer caution against books and music, but the pay gap and the continuing lack of women at the top of the corporate ladder shows that the idea of innate female weakness is still having its malign effects.

Being keen on sex could be very bad for your health

When it came to sex, too much stimulation was also seriously harmful, leading to nymphomania and masturbation, but so also was too little. Surprisingly, the treatment for too little was genital massage. This eventually resulted in an invention, impossible to reconcile with our stereotype of strait-laced Victorian ladies, of steam-powered vibrators to relieve the doctors' tired hands.

But it was not all a matter of discreet relief of sexual urges.

---

2   Henry Maudsley 'Sex in Mind and in Education', *Fortnightly Review*, new series, 15 April 1874, 466–83.

Too much sex was treated far more brutally – with what we now call female genital mutilation (FGM). In asylums around the country, special surgeries were set up where nymphomania and other manifestations of hysteria were treated with cauterising or cutting off the clitoris.

Removal of the ovaries or removal of the womb altogether was another treatment, deemed a humane mercy for women with any form of mental instability. There are estimates that over 100,000 women were 'de-sexed' in this way. And again, as we have seen, the hysterectomy is still considered an acceptable treatment for such 'women's problems' as excessive monthly bleeding.

What these mostly worthy, intelligent medical men were missing when connecting the disorders with either the body or the mind was, as we now know, an understanding of hormones and their importance for both. For over a hundred years, knowledge has been growing about how this complex interaction works, but for so much of that time, women have been the victims of their hormones.

Marilyn Monroe: sex goddess who suffered for it

So why do we continue to allow this to be the case? This is the twenty-first century and we have the knowledge to help. Sometimes I wonder if we have the will. We know that an imbalance of our hormones puts us mentally and physically out of kilter. If we accept that hormones play a large part in our health and well-being, then why is it not a more ubiquitous route to treatment?

There are so many women who suffer from all sorts of psychological and psychiatric health problems, from mood swings to depression, anxiety and panic attacks, and even illness as severe as psychosis. Many could find relief, if not the solution to their woes, if they had a well-balanced hormonal system.

Marilyn Monroe is a classic example. She might have been one of the many who could have been helped in the last century had her hormonal situation been properly addressed. She suffered not only psychologically, but also physically.

On 5 August 1962, the banner headline in the *LA Times* screamed: 'Marilyn Monroe found dead'; Marilyn, the biggest star in Hollywood, had died at the age of thirty-six from an overdose of sleeping pills, and suicide was suspected.

Superficially she had everything to live for. She was at the peak of her career, with twenty-four movies to her name. She had experienced a meteoric rise from humble origins to become the most marketable film star of her time, and even today her name is synonymous with sex appeal. How had this fairy tale ended in tragedy?

What we do know is that Marilyn was a deeply unhappy and hormonally unbalanced woman – and she had been this way for her whole life. Born Norma Jeane Mortenson in June 1926, she was the illegitimate child of an unstable mother who was hospitalised shortly after her birth and went on to suffer repeated mental breakdowns. So little Norma Jeane had a chaotic childhood, in and out of orphanages and boarding with a series of foster parents. In later life, she said that one foster father had raped her when she was eight. She was sexually active early, marrying a boy from her neighbourhood at the age of sixteen.

Dreams of stardom became a reality when, two years later, with her husband away at war, she took to modelling and was discovered by a photographer, who propelled her into the Hollywood milieu. Her looks, her platinum-blonde hair and hourglass figure, became her passport to fame and fortune.

She was, by all accounts, a woman of many facets: mercurial, temperamental, volatile, easily slighted, sometimes aggressive and perennially late on set. She was plagued with doubts about her ability and was dependent on acting coaches to boost her confidence.

During the 1950s, Marilyn was the darling of the gossip columns and lived her life in the spotlight, divorcing three times. Her second husband, world-famous baseball player Joe DiMaggio, was followed in 1956 by the king of New York intellectuals, avant-garde playwright Arthur Miller. The contrast was captured by *Variety* magazine's caption: 'Egghead weds Hourglass'.

Some people said she was a frigid iceberg in bed, others that she was highly sexed. She certainly had a number of high-profile affairs with co-stars including Yves Montand and Tony Curtis, and more than likely with both Robert and John Kennedy.

Vulnerable and impulsive, she was in fact a highly intelligent woman who tried to control her career by taking on the movie moguls and setting up her own production company; she was apparently frustrated with her 'sex goddess' image and wanted to be taken seriously, as her last two movies, both highbrow, indicate.

Yet underneath this veneer of glamour and glitz lies a murky tale of sadness and despair. We know she was keen to have children, but she suffered from painful endometriosis all her life. She had at least three miscarriages. She was an insomniac and gradually became dependent on cocktails of sleeping pills, barbiturates, painkillers and alcohol.

As her marriage to Miller broke down in the humiliating glare of publicity, she collapsed and spent early 1961 battling with ill health. She had surgery for her endometriosis and spent a month in hospital recuperating and having treatment for depression.

At the time of her death she was veering between high hopes of success for her next film – a biopic of Jean Harlow, a Hollywood legend who had died tragically early at the age of twenty-six – and complete unreliability on the set of the one she was currently shooting. The movie company sacked her but then reinstated her in July. A few weeks later, she was dead.

With hindsight, we can say that mentally and physically the odds were against her. Her curvy, bosomy figure plus her endometriosis strongly suggest she was suffering from high oestrogen dominance (a prime cause of endometriosis), along with severe fluctuations in progesterone levels.

She may also have suffered from bipolar disorder, inherited from her mother, which often goes hand in hand with hormonal imbalances. We can only speculate how different Marilyn's story might have been if the many experts and psychiatrists she depended on had known about how hormones can compound our misery when they are allowed to get completely out of balance.

No doubt the drinking and the pills didn't help, and she was definitely depressed, but did she mean to kill herself, or just want some respite from the 'black dog' of despair and insomnia exacerbated by her hormones?

If Marilyn had been my patient, I would have taken careful note of her history. She had a very difficult start, not only socially but also genetically. Daughters can often take after their mothers, and hers had had a hard life as well as being mentally quite unstable and suffering from postnatal depression.

Marilyn's high oestrogen levels would have benefited from progesterone's calming effect, which could well have lessened her anxiety and depression, as well as reducing the frequent pain of endometriosis and possibly even helping her to maintain a viable pregnancy.

Controlling attitudes to women that still persist

There is a long history of regarding women as 'unhinged' when they try to express their creativity, emotions or intelligence in ways that are considered unpredictable. It's awful to imagine what would have been in store for Marilyn – with her sexual magnetism and behaviour that would have been diagnosed as hysterical – had she been committed to a Victorian asylum.

The direct brutality is gone, but the impact of the assumptions behind it persisted into the last century and have become entrenched in social attitudes and stereotypes that continue to this day. 'Women's problems' are still often regarded as a colossal joke and used as an excuse to keep women from excelling, to sell them more products and to make them pay more for them (think of the tampon tax!).

I'd like you to know that you are not alone with what is happening to you. Women through the centuries have suffered and continue to suffer the consequences of hormones in disarray. The way you feel can seem overwhelming, taking over your mood, actions and behaviour. It is irrational and to the outside world does not make any sense. We who suffer from hormonal imbalance do not understand what is happening. We no longer feel as if we are in control, because our hormones are controlling us.

True as this is, it immediately raises another issue that I know will trouble some of you. Women have spent three generations trying to establish themselves as equals to men, and we still find ourselves in a world where men frequently dominate the agenda. We rightly want to be accepted as of equal value, with equal opportunities for advancement in careers and pay, sharing the responsibilities of child-rearing with our chosen mates, or indeed choosing to be a sole parent.

As a result, if we accept the view that there really are differences between the male and female mind, initiated by differing bodily processes and reactions, then surely we play into the hands of those entrenched patriarchal forces who want to keep women 'in their place' – in the home, making babies and cherry pies.

I am the last person in the world to advocate such an outcome. I was brought up fighting for the rights of women. But equally I will not be cowed by political correctness into denying what I know to be the case. Women are not asking for special treatment, but the world has moved on. We are no longer confined to bed as treatment for that mysterious, fantastical condition hysteria. The idea that there is an inherent female weakness that prevents us taking our rightful place in the world on an equal footing with men is archaic and should be abandoned. Far from hindering us, our womanhood is a source of strength.

We know that hormone replacement, using bio-identical supplements, is a simple and effective response to deal with any imbalance in those now not so mysterious chemical messengers. Symptoms such as headaches, premenstrual tension, sleep disturbance, mood swings and the inevitable menopause may have a day-to-day impact on our lives, but if we take control of what is happening to us, we will no longer need to, nor should we have to, put up with them.

The problems that come with being unable to make the hormone insulin – i.e. diabetes – can be even more serious than some other hormonal dysfunctions, yet we don't consider that needing insulin replacement therapy disqualifies diabetics from doing anything.

What we need is a new approach. One that accepts the reality of our hormones, understands their significance, empowers us to choose what is going to work best for us and deals head-on with any problems caused by imbalance. We cannot deny the reality of biology, but if we understand it, we can work with it rather than having it work against us.

We need to understand what is happening so that we can help ourselves.

The protocols I've outlined in this book will help when we suffer symptoms that are foreign to us or that have become exacerbated. We no longer have to reach for the antidepressants we were prescribed for our anxiety or fatigue or low mood or insomnia. There are bio-identical hormones for hormone balancing or replacement, mood foods to enhance and calm our neurotransmitters, supplements and herbs that will help improve our brain chemistry and resolve our symptoms. Lifestyle changes, mindfulness and any other stress-reducing pursuits will complement what we are doing, so that we can feel like ourselves again.

SUMMARY OF KEY POINTS

- Women now have greater control over sex and fertility but at the risk of denying the value of their hormonal rhythms.
- Brutal Victorian madhouses are gone, but echoes of the attitudes behind them still linger on.
- Modern medical research has often excluded women from drug trials because hormonal changes can mess up the results,

increasing the risk that women will suffer side effects when the drug goes to market.

- Less interference in women's minds and bodies by official organisations and medical men in the past might have reduced the inequalities that still exist.
- An overview of Victorian-style control of females reveals where inequalities originated.
- A popular explanation for female emotional distress was the 'wandering womb', which sent them mad.
- The 'madness' women could suffer following childbirth was described in the early nineteenth century. It is still not treated well today.
- Freud shifted attention from physical to mental and unconscious causes of madness.
- Was there a connection between increasing diagnosis of madness and the growing demands from women to be taken seriously?
- Books and music were said to be too stimulating for sensitive women.
- Because woman were 'sick' for a week every month, it was believed that they were unfit for hard work. An echo of this is found in the continuing pay gap.
- Having too much or too little sex was considered bad for women's health.
- Sexually active women diagnosed with nymphomania were treated punitively with FGM or de-sexed with a hysterectomy.
- Women can still be penalised for overt sexuality and erratic

hormonal behaviour. Marilyn Monroe was one of these. We know enough to treat women more effectively now.

- Marilyn had a magnetic screen presence and an erratic and unstable personal life. Her voluptuous figure plus endometriosis suggest her oestrogen levels were unbalanced and she lacked sufficient progesterone. With proper hormonal treatment her life might have been much more fulfilled and happy.
- Women no longer need to suffer the social consequences of having hormones in disarray.
- Acknowledging the benefit of hormone replacement does not indicate weakness any more than needing the hormone insulin disqualifies anyone with diabetes from a challenging career.

CHAPTER EIGHT

OUR TOXIC ENVIRONMENT

● ● ● ●

It's now well known that our environment – the air, the sea, water supplies – contains a vast variety of potent new chemical compounds, such as pesticides, food additives and industrial materials, some of which can fool our bodies into treating them as natural hormones. Just as the artificial hormones used in HRT and the like can have different and damaging effects not found with bio-identicals, the 'hormone disrupters', as they are known, can cause problems of their own, though these are far more wide-ranging and serious.

The sheer number of these new chemicals – 80,000 created since 1945 – is surprising and alarming, as is the disruption they can cause in our bodies. They are found in many of the everyday objects that surround us, such as plastics, cosmetics, paints, furniture, electronics and even food; their effects include changing the levels of various hormones (possibly by turning one hormone into another), interfering with the signals our natural hormones are delivering – such as instructing cells to die early – and being stored in our organs.

Our endocrine system connects and manages insulin, oestrogen, progesterone and testosterone, which are produced by glands that have effects all around the body and brain – the pituitary, thyroid, adrenal, ovaries and testicles. Thus the potential effect of hormone disrupters is huge. We are talking about interfering with important functions such as growth, reproduction, blood pressure and the immediate use we make of our food – whether we store it or use it for energy.

Regulators have been slow to react

If all that wasn't seriously worrying enough, the risks have been known for decades and yet there is still no real attention being paid to the long-term impact of these substances. There is no requirement to prove they are safe *before* use, although there is a requirement to prove them unsafe *after* use. But how we are to do this without impacting our health and well-being as a society is unclear.

Sure, national and international regulating bodies have attempted to keep up, but they are hampered by conflicts of interest and a lack of resources. In my view, the unintended consequences will only become fully evident in our children's children – they are the ones most at risk. Reproductive problems and diseases such as cancer are on the rise, whilst our children's cognitive development and IQ is apparently on the decline. Are we happy being part of an enormous global experiment?

Amongst the long list of chemicals invented since the Second World War, one of the hormone disrupters that really concerns me is bisphenol A (BPA), which is a xeno-estrogen, meaning that the body responds to it as if it was oestrogen. It has been used commercially since 1957 in the manufacture of polycarbonate, a lightweight, tough, transparent plastic that is widely used because it is easily worked and moulded. Alarm bells have been ringing about its safety since 1997, after research showed it could disrupt normal development in animal foetuses, but industry has continued to use it prolifically for a wide range of products, from containers to children's toys.

Scientists can't agree about the dangers

By 2004, risks to humans from BPA were showing up in reports suggesting that exposure was 'associated with higher levels of anxiety, depression, hyperactivity and aggression in children', and the US National Institute of Health determined that it had 'some concerns' about effects on foetal and infant brain development and behaviour.[1]

And yet not only can BPA still be found in plastic containers, baby bottles, water bottles and plastic bags, it is even in the epoxy resin lining of drinks cans, dental filling sealants, household electronics, spectacle lenses, plastic piping and children's toys. Paper recycled into children's books and cash till receipts is coated in it. When you microwave your baby's bottle, or let your child chew the corner of their new book, or collect bundles of till receipts, you are exposing yourself and your family to a harmful chemical with potential long-term effects. Between the 1980s and 2009, the world production of BPA more than doubled to 2.2 million tonnes.

The failure to take effective steps to deal with the possible risks of BPA shows clearly why hormone disrupters are so difficult to deal with. A major stumbling block is that scientists can't agree on the risks or how great they are. The European Food Safety Authority (EFSA) says: 'BPA poses no health risk to consumers of any age group (including unborn children, infants and adolescents) at

---

1   https://www.ncbi.nlm.nih.gov/pmc/articles/PMC2799471/

current exposure levels.' On the other hand, in 2017 the European Chemicals Agency said that BPA should be listed as a 'substance of very high concern'.[2] [3]

How BPA sows confusion among the hormones

BPA is undoubtedly an oestrogen mimic, which means that it will influence the actions of oestrogen in the body. As we have seen time and time again, it can be very damaging when the balance between oestrogen and other hormones is disturbed. Have a look at this diagram of a BPA molecule compared with one of oestrogen and you will see that its shape and form is a 'chemical lookalike' and it can behave like an oestradiol molecule and disrupt normal oestrogen activity.

BISPHENOL A

OESTRADIOL

---

2   M. Ejaredar et al., 'Bisphenol A exposure and children's behavior: A systematic review', *Journal of Exposure Science & Environmental Epidemiology*, March 2016. Available at: doi:10.1038/jes.2016.8. PMID 26956939.

3   https://echa.europa.eu/hot-topics/bisphenol-a

When BPA gets into your body, it will sit on your oestrogen receptors and switch them on. The result will be that your body becomes confused about how much natural oestrogen to produce. What's more, your other hormones struggle to deal effectively with this interloper. Is it friend or foe? Over time, your endocrine system will become compromised.

So if BPA is known to be a powerful hormone disrupter, how come the regulators don't demand manufacturers take special care? The answer illustrates another stumbling block to effective regulation. BPA was never supposed to get into our food chain, so the safety tests it is required to pass are nowhere near as stringent as those applied to our food. There is no requirement to list it as an ingredient anywhere, even though we now know it leaches into our food and water as it breaks down and finds its way into all corners of our lives. We have no choice about our exposure to it because we don't know it's there.

And what about the risk to the foetus?

BPA doesn't just show up in food. Over twenty years ago, experiments on animals found that foetuses can be damaged by exposure to it from the earliest stage of pregnancy. So could it cause defects in your unborn baby? Your placenta is designed to filter out harmful toxins, and it does a pretty good job, but BPA still gets through. The problem is that we can't do the sort of experiments necessary on humans, for good reasons.

What this means is that nothing will be done, given the commercial pressures to continue with BPA's use, until the impact is so obvious it can't be ignored. And that means, under the current regime, watching and waiting for several generations before acting. BPA has a short life span and our systems can detoxify low exposures, but do we really want to wait decades to find out what happens to ourselves or our children?

Even low levels of chemical exposure can affect brain development in unborn and young children. Population studies in the USA show a downwards shift in the average youth IQ. The long-term consequences of using our children as human guinea pigs will be profound.

Disrupters at work?

It is worrying enough that developmental problems related to disrupters may be showing up in future generations, but young men already have a problem. There has been a steep rise in a condition known as testicular dysgenesis syndrome, a disorder that involves a cluster of developmental failings in the womb.

These include the penis not developing properly (hypospadias), undescended testicles (cryptorchidism), poor-quality semen and testicular cancer. A poorly developed penis is now the second most common birth defect in male babies in the UK, affecting one in every 250 boys; meanwhile, worldwide, 40 per cent of young males have low sperm count, while the fertility rate in those under thirty has decreased by 15 per cent.

This is no surprise. Sperm is designed for one thing only: to find and fertilise a female egg. It is too small to have built-in protection against toxins and is extremely vulnerable to external influences. If sperm is exposed to toxins while it is being made, it is likely that it will be damaged. These changes are happening too fast to be genetic; they must be environmental. But how can we prove the harm exposure to disrupters is doing?

Not just fertility is being affected; cancers and hormonal disorders are on the increase too. Over the last thirty years, testicular cancer in Australia has risen by over 50 per cent. In the UK, the incidence is up 30 per cent since 1993. Between 1975 and 2012, all adolescent cancers in the USA increased by 25 per cent, but testicular and thyroid cancer increased the most.

As doctors, we know something is going on, we know that there is an 'effect' from somewhere, but where? Could it come from the disrupting hormones that are all around us?

Maybe. Researchers have found that if you give pregnant rats chemicals that block testosterone production (anti-androgens) or raise oestrogen levels, the penises and testicles of their male pups don't develop properly, and if they do father any pups themselves, those pups are likely to be less fertile. The pups can also develop cancers in the cells that make hormones, such as the adrenals, as well as those making chemical messengers (neurotransmitters such as serotonin) in the brain. This has a devastating effect on mood and behaviour. But it is obviously impossible to run experiments to prove this happens in humans.

It's not only our sons who are suffering or will suffer in the future. Our daughters can also be severely impacted by these hormone disrupters. A report from the Endocrine Society in the USA recently updated the evidence for endocrine-related disorders and found the average age of puberty in females had come down from twelve to nine. [4]

This is no surprise either. As I described in Chapter One, female puberty is stimulated by a shot of oestrogen into the system. We

---

4   'Secondary sexual characteristics and menses in young girls seen in office practice: a study from the Pediatric Research in Office Settings network', 1997 Apr; 99(4):505-12, https://www.ncbi.nlm.nih.gov/pubmed/9093289

know that hormones only require minute doses to have a biological effect. If you give oestrogen to very young female rats, they come into puberty: it is logical that humans under the influence of disrupters might well do the same – but it can't be proven, so we continue to ignore it![5] Early puberty can cause physical and emotional problems in children. Young girls will experience early breast development and will stop growing. Short stature is frequently the outcome. Early puberty is experienced physically before the brain can deal with the changes. On an emotional level, some children can become sexually active at a younger age, and this can lead to addiction problems like eating disorders.

More couples can't conceive

So far, we've been focusing on the effects of endocrine disruption in the womb and childhood, but of course the impact on us is lifelong. Couples experiencing infertility problems, for example, go through their own private hell, but are they also part of a larger and growing problem? Approximately 10 per cent of couples in the United States are defined as infertile based on their inability to conceive after twelve months of unprotected intercourse, while one in seven couples in the UK have difficulty conceiving. There is a strong likelihood that disrupters are involved there too. Are we really willing to continue compromising our fertility to fuel the never-ending boom in commercialised chemicals?

There are plenty of other hidden sources of these chemicals.

---

5   Dina Fine Maron, 'Why Girls are starting Puberty Early', *Scientific American*, May 2015, 312, 5.

Did you know that they are now responsible for nearly 50 per cent of toxins in the air we breathe? Chemicals in perfume and air fresheners are designed to evaporate into the air. Our atmosphere is pervaded by these harmful micro particles, and we, as consumers, are demanding more and more of them.

Disrupters at work in your home

Many of these disrupters are petroleum derivatives but unlike gasoline itself, they are not contained in storage tanks. Instead the disrupting chemicals in pesticides, cleaning products, printing ink, adhesives, soaps and detergents all spread freely through the environment.

And the effects can be alarmingly specific. Flame retardants, found in a variety of products around us, such as plastics, paint, furniture, electronics and even food, contain a dopamine-type chemical that interferes with the development of the frontal cortex – the area of the brain that manages impulse control and quick thinking.

Perhaps even more pervasive are the parabens, another oestrogen lookalike, that are added to cosmetics as a preservative. The European Commission on Endocrine Disruption lists them as a 'Category 1' – meaning there is good evidence for their effect on animal hormone function. Parabens have been detected in human breast cancer tissue and have been found to interfere with our nervous, immune and reproductive systems.

Yet we continue to plaster beauty products on our faces and bodies, largely unaware of the effect they are having because, sadly, cosmetic companies do not need to list ingredients with much precision, on the grounds that they are not intended for human consumption. This is despite the fact that research has shown that many of these chemicals penetrate the skin and build up a presence in the blood.

The disrupters lurking in cosmetics are not limited to parabens. Another culprit is a family of chemicals called phthalates, which are 'plasticisers', meaning they make plastics flexible. In 2008, a National Health survey in the US warned of the danger of high levels of phthalate exposure in the adult population.[6]

Phthalates are a known oestrogen disrupter, and numerous studies have shown they cause reproductive abnormalities in animals and humans, and are linked to decreased testosterone production in boys, fertility problems, endometriosis in women, premature delivery of babies, asthma and skin allergies.

The National Health survey found that women had higher levels of phthalates than men, no doubt due to their more pervasive use of shampoos, cosmetics and creams. Most effective at getting phthalates into the bloodstream were nail polish, hairspray and perfume, because the compounds help the products to cling to your skin and hair. And exposure starts young. Babies tested in the same survey showed high levels of phthalates in their urine from all those specialised baby powders and lotions.

But phthalates are not just used in cosmetics; they are also found in the likes of packaging, cling film, detergents, vinyl floor covering, and lubricating oils. Do we really want them surrounding us? A study published in *Environmental Health Perspectives* even looked at the relation between phthalates in urine and insulin resistance, connecting endocrine disorders such as diabetes

---

6   https://wwwn.cdc.gov/Nchs/Nhanes/2003-2004/L24PH_C.htm

to phthalate levels and asking the question, 'Could exposure to these chemicals be linked to the obesity epidemic?'[7]

Loopholes in the regulations

The phthalate problem has been known about and studied for nearly twenty years, so why are these chemicals still so ubiquitous? Are we mad? Sadly, the solution is not as simple as just pointing out that a compound, even ones as widespread as phthalates or BPA, can cause all sorts of hormonal havoc. When this happens and the risks becomes widely publicised, companies jump on the bandwagon and bring out BPA-free or phthalate-free products. But beware, as these often contain substitutes just as harmful but which have not yet been tested in the global 'experiment'.

You might think the consumer goods companies would make efforts to find harmless alternatives, but sadly, if problems arise, they can get around them by substituting other substances that have yet to be listed as potentially dangerous compounds. Ultimately it will be pressure from consumers that will change the ways of chemical companies. After all, the companies want to sell their wares, and with our new-found awareness, we can demand what is safe for us and our environment.

These disrupters have insinuated themselves so successfully into our domestic lives due to a failure of effective regulation. It's very clear to me that there is an inherent conflict of interest when

---

7   Richard W. Stahlhut, 'Concentrations of Urinary Phthalate Metabolites are Associated with Increased Waist Circumference and Insulin Resistance in Adult US Males', *Environmental Health Perspectives*, June 2007, 115(6), 876–82. Available at: http://www.ncbi.nlm.nih.gov/pmc/articles/ PMC1892109/?tool=pmcentrez.

companies that make a product are expected to test it for safety themselves, and their recommendations are then used as the basis for working out regulations on safe levels of exposure. Politics and profit get in the way.

For example, in 2014, the French government put in place a ban on BPA in paper products, but found that the companies simply replaced it with other forms of bisphenol – BPS or BPB, which are similar but have little or no data behind them. Industry lobbyists are now hard at work attempting to overturn the ban, whilst regulators are attempting to uphold it. Recently the EFSA has lowered the BPA levels considered safe from 50mg to 4mg, but in reality, research shows that our brains, breasts, prostates and thyroids are all affected by minute amounts of hormone disrupters. There is no safe level!

And even when one chemical is flagged as potentially harmful and subjected to tests and greater regulatory control, the reality is that most consumer goods contain a cocktail of these chemicals – a challenge that is proving too tough for regulators to police when they have meagre budgets and are answerable to their political masters.

Lifestyle changes that can help protect you

What, then, are we to do to combat this unseen invasion of chemical toxins that have permeated into every corner of our homes and lives? Making changes to our lifestyle is one place to start. At the very least, we can follow those well-known but often ignored admonitions to wash all fruit and vegetables, buy organic produce, give up canned goods and convenience foods and stop using commercially produced make-up, shampoo and cleaning products.

The Amish, the American sect who follow such rules, have significantly lower levels of BPA and phthalates in their systems, but it is not realistic to expect mainstream society to change its habits so drastically. What we do need to do is lobby for national and international regulations to have proper teeth, to be globally enforced and not to be subverted by political or commercial expediency.

Public pressure and political will needed

We know progress can be made when there is a concerted will to change. Pressure on politicians has eventually brought about changes in areas such as banning smoking and leaded petrol. Efforts to lower dangerous emissions of lead and mercury from industrial plants and cars have had measurable positive results.

There have been some significant developments in protecting our environment and ourselves. In 2004, the Stockholm Convention was signed, ratifying an international treaty restricting 'chemicals with known impacts on human health'. It listed the 'dirty dozen' worst chemicals banned from use, which included DDT (dichlorodiphenyltrichloroethane) and PCB (polychlorinated biphenyls). Both these chemicals are neurotoxins, and had over time caused serious damage to those exposed to them, including cancers, miscarriage, thyroid and liver disease and immune problems. The impact of these chemical pollutants will persist for generations, but at least the legislation made further cases much less likely.

So there is some good news amongst the gloom. Since DDT was banned in the USA in the 1970s, tests have shown marked reductions in blood levels in human and animal populations, though it is still present in the oceans, the soil and the atmosphere.

The smoking debate lasted for decades before we were galvanised into action, with the forces of corporate lobbyists ranged against the health professionals, but eventually sanity prevailed and smoking is down 20 per cent, with the incidence of lung cancer finally slowing. So we know that regulation does work when implemented effectively, and we are starting to wake up to the damage we are doing not only to ourselves but to the world around us.

Our children won't forgive us if we stay silent. I am heartened by the recent surge of activism against the scourge of plastics contaminating our environment and the oceans, and hope this is the beginning of a sea change in awareness and empowerment – we must not wait until it is too late. There is no possible benefit from having these toxic hormonal disrupters in our bodies, so let's make it impossible for them to get there!

SUMMARY OF KEY POINTS

- Since the Second World War, 80,000 new and potentially dangerous chemical compounds have been made.
- Many of these find their way into our environment – food, water, cosmetics – and can disrupt our hormones.
- Although the risks have been known for decades, very little has been done – cancers and reproductive issues are on the rise, and IQs are lowering.
- BPA is an especially worrying compound that is used widely.
- Scientists can't agree on the dangers, confusing the message.
- BPA can mimic oestrogen, causing disruption to our natural

hormones and compromising the endocrine system.

- BPA has been shown to pose a risk to animal foetuses, but it is impossible to do the same experiments on humans, and so the risks go mostly ignored.
- Hormone disrupters can affect the development of male genitalia – testicular dysgenesis syndrome – and are affecting male fertility.
- More couples can't conceive: 1 in 10 in America and 1 in 7 in the UK.
- Hormone disrupters are especially prevalent in cosmetics, and can pass through the skin.
- There are loopholes in regulations that allow manufacturers to replace one harmful chemical with another.
- There are some lifestyle changes that can protect you, but these are difficult in modern life.
- The way to change the amount of toxins we're exposed to is through pressuring our political institutions and calling for change.

CHAPTER NINE

HOW TO HELP YOURSELF

● ● ● ●

I wrote this book in the hope of creating greater awareness about the importance of our hormones, in terms of both how they function and how they affect our daily lives.

We know that mental health is highly complex and can be attributed to many causes, and in my belief it should be treated by looking at both the mind and the body. Physiological impacts are now being increasingly recognised as having a role in mental health symptoms. Hormones are one of these impacts, and for many a very significant factor.

My purpose throughout this book is to arm you with everything you need to know, so that no one has to suffer needlessly as a result of hormone imbalance. I want you to realise that you are not alone in what you are experiencing, and that you can implement what you've learnt to improve your general well-being.

I have always believed that responsibility for your hormonal health sits with you yourself, and not just with your doctor. An understanding of how hormones work and their effects should not be confined to the medical realm. Everyone has hormones and therefore everyone should know how to manage them. Hormone imbalance symptoms such as headaches, premenstrual tension, sleep disturbance, mood swings and the inevitable menopause are all part of life. The knowledge of why you experience these things is powerful in its own right. But we can take it one step further, by taking control of our hormones instead of allowing them to take control of us.

In this chapter I set out a practical guide on how to help yourself when you realise that you may be having specific hormonal issues, be it during puberty, pregnancy or menopause. It's also intended for people without specific hormone complaints who nonetheless want to safeguard their hormonal health and well-being. These suggestions deal with everything other than hormone replacement therapy. HRT is just one tool in our arsenal, but it shouldn't be the only one. Diet, exercise, sleep, environment and stress play important roles, and any hormone intervention that ignores these factors is incomplete.

Before we start, I want to once again articulate the ethos behind how I practise medicine – an ethos that also drives the suggestions contained in this chapter. I believe first and foremost that we must accept the reality of our hormones and understand their significance in our lives. This will hopefully empower us to choose what steps we take to address any imbalance. In short: we cannot deny the reality of biology, but if we understand it, we can work with it rather than have it work against us.

Lifestyle changes

There is no denying the power of lifestyle to either make or break your general well-being. There are many simple things we can do to resolve or minimise the effects of stressors in our lives and environment as well as the hormonal changes taking place in our bodies at the various stages of life. I have always advocated lifestyle and nutrition as a starting point, and this chapter is all about giving you some simple protocols to follow.

Diet

What hasn't already been written about the importance of our diet for our well-being? Very little. I cannot hope in this short chapter to make even a tiny dent in the enormous body of complex, often contradictory knowledge about how to improve one's health through diet. Here I will summarize and reiterate what I have already advocated in previous chapters and share the few things that I have come to believe over forty years of working with people to help them feel better.

Below are lists of foods I believe you should try to include in your diet. I certainly do. I don't make any recommendations about how much of them you should eat or in what ratios. Enough books have been written on that topic. For each group I provide a short explanation of why you should eat these foods and what role they play.

Carbohydrates

There are two types of carbohydrates: simple and complex. The difference between the two is the amount of sugar molecules each carbohydrate comprises and how fast those sugar molecules are absorbed into our system.

Complex carbohydrates are made up of hundreds of sugar molecules and also tend to be packed with fibre and nutrients such as vitamins, minerals and antioxidants. The sugars in complex carbohydrates are absorbed and digested much more slowly into our system. This means that we receive a consistent supply of slow-release glucose to the brain, keeping us clearly focused and boosting our brain function.

Simple carbohydrates are made up of only a few sugar molecules and are digested and absorbed much more quickly into our bloodstream and brain. As a result, the brain can receive a short-term high – what we call a 'sugar hit'. Unfortunately, the effect is only short-lived, and afterwards you can feel tired, fuzzy-brained and hungry.

Carbohydrates to include in your diet:

- oatmeal
- brown rice
- sweet potato and yams
- multigrain cereal (barley, oats and rye)
- white potato with skins
- wholewheat bread
- wholewheat pasta
- beans and lentils
- couscous
- quinoa
- beets
- butternut squash
- pumpkin

Vegetables

Vegetables are special in that they often have incredibly high nutrient value compared to other kinds of foods. Many vegetables are rich in vitamin A, as well as B vitamins such as B1 (thiamine), B2 (riboflavin), B3 (niacin), B5 (pantothenic acid), B6 (pyridoxine), folic acid and vitamin B12 (cobalamin). They are also a good source of vitamin C, vitamin E and vitamin K, as well as minerals such as potassium, calcium, phosphorus, magnesium, zinc, copper, manganese, selenium and chromium.

Vegetables to include in your diet:

- broccoli
- kale
- asparagus
- spinach
- salad greens
- tomatoes
- peppers
- onion
- mushrooms
- cucumber
- courgettes
- carrots
- green beans
- peas
- cauliflower

Fats

In our diet-mad world, fats are often seen as the enemy. But the truth is that we really cannot live a healthy, balanced life without them. Fats are a source and storage box of energy. They are also the building blocks of all cellular membranes and of steroid hormones. Restrict your intake of fats too much, and you risk cutting off your body's ability to manufacture hormones. Essential fats are also an integral part of our brain and the myelin sheath that surrounds the nerve cells. Additionally, they are important for the absorption of fat-soluble vitamins such as A, D, E and K, and for healthy skin tissue. We starve ourselves of fats at our peril.

Healthy sources of good fats to include in your diet:

- flaxseed/linseed
- almonds
- olive oil
- avocado
- walnuts
- virgin coconut oil
- wild salmon
- peanuts
- ghee (clarified butter)
- peanut oil
- olives
- hemp seed oil
- pecan
- cashews
- dark chocolate

Protein

Be sure not to ignore protein. It is needed for the repair, growth and maintenance of all the body's tissues and cells. In other words, proteins maintain the body's muscles, bones and organs. Like fats and carbohydrates, proteins can also act as a source of energy for the body.

Proteins to include in your diet:

- eggs
- organic poultry

- turkey breast
- wild salmon
- canned tuna
- nuts (walnuts, almonds, pecans)
- pumpkin
- sesame seeds
- organic beef
- tofu
- Greek yoghurt
- cod fish
- rainbow trout

Vitamins, minerals and herbs

Food is where you'll get most of your nutrients, but depending on your diet and your specific needs, it might not be enough. There are a multitude of vitamins, herbs and minerals we can take. Below is a short list of what I consider the 'greatest hits' that we really need in order to make sure our mood, mind and vitality are well looked after.

Fatty acids

Omega-3 essential fatty acids come from cold-water fish. Fish oils can enhance memory and the cellular communication and actions of neurotransmitters. An inadequate supply of essential omega-3 fatty acids may be a factor in developing depression.

Omega-6 essential fatty acids (linoleic acid) come from flaxseed, pumpkin and sunflower seeds. Grapeseed oil, evening primrose oil and borage oil are all good sources of omega-6 and should be included in the food you eat. Omega-6 can be converted in the body to prostaglandins, which are hormone-like substances that contribute to hormone production and nerve transmission. GLA from evening primrose oil and borage oil has been shown to improve many premenstrual symptoms, including headaches, depression, irritability and bloating. It is recommended to take omega-3 with omega-6 for PMS symptoms.

Vitamins

Vitamins A, C and E are primary antioxidants and are readily found in your diet. Antioxidants protect the cells in your body from the effects of free radicals, which are molecules produced by our bodies when we break down food or are exposed to toxins such as pollution, smoke or radiation.

B vitamins are vital for stress tolerance as well as essential for proper nervous system function. They also help in unlocking energy from the food you eat. B vitamin deficiencies are often associated with anxiety and nervous disorders. **Vitamin B6** is required for hormonal balance. It is involved in brain chemistry and nervous system function. Scientific studies have proven its effectiveness in the prevention of PMS symptoms.

Vitamin E may be beneficial in addressing nervousness and depression.

Vitamin D is the only vitamin that is actually a hormone. Vitamin D deficiency may be a contributor to depressive symptoms that occur during the winter. The lack of sunshine coinciding with a drop in vitamin D may affect serotonin levels in the brain. Vitamin D also helps calcium absorption for the bones.

Minerals

Magnesium is a smooth muscle relaxant and has a calming effect on nerves. It is needed to balance neurotransmitters in the brain and to alleviate mood swings. Magnesium plays a key role in the regulation of many hormones and neurotransmitters. It is one of the essential minerals to make serotonin. It reduces stress hormones and is vital for a good night's sleep.

Calcium together with magnesium is needed for the proper function of muscles and nerves. Deficiencies in these minerals may lead to irritability, tension and insomnia.

Zinc is an essential trace element for healthy brain function and immunity.

Selenium is an important micronutrient for the brain and thyroid function. It is also an important antioxidant.

Amino acids

L-theanine is a wonderful amino acid that calms you down without sedating you. Theanine crosses the blood–brain barrier and may have an influence on the neurotransmitters serotonin and dopamine.

Methionine may facilitate the removal of excessive oestrogen in the body through a process called methylation, which takes place in the liver. The best results are achieved if methionine is combined with vitamin B6 and fibre to remove oestrogen via the gut. A lot of PMS symptoms can also be attributed to elevated oestrogen levels.

Tryptophan is the amino acid that is necessary to produce 5-HTP, the precursor to serotonin. 5-HTP is also a precursor to melatonin, the brain hormone that helps us sleep.

Tyrosine is an amino acid that is essential for the synthesis of thyroid hormones. It is also necessary for the formation of adrenaline and noradrenaline by the adrenal glands. This is one of the reasons why adrenal fatigue can impact your thyroid function.

Herbs

Rhodiola, also known as arctic or golden root, helps balance cortisol levels. It can enhance the transport of serotonin precursors such as tryptophan and 5-HTP into the brain. This in turn increases serotonin activity in the brain.

Siberian ginseng increases our tolerance and response to stress, be it mental, physical or environmental. It can help in the production and regulation of adrenal gland hormones. It supports adrenal function, which is very important for those suffering from chronic stress.

Ginkgo biloba (maidenhair tree) is beneficial in improving memory and cognitive function, positive mood and increased energy. It works by enhancing the brain's microcirculation and utilising glucose and oxygen in the brain cells.

Dong quai (*Angelica sinensis*) is also known as 'female ginseng'. It is one of the most widely taken female tonics and is commonly used for menopausal symptoms. Dong quai may have an oestrogen-regulating effect and can relieve hot flushes, palpitations and irritability.

St John's wort (*Hypericum perforatum*) has been scientifically proven to relieve mild to moderate depression. It may also improve mood swings, relieve anxiety and reduce symptoms of premenstrual tension. St John's wort should not be used together with SSRIs or any other antidepressants that increase serotonin. Too much serotonin can have deleterious side effects.

Feverfew is a flowering plant from the daisy family. Ingesting feverfew can reduce the frequency of migraine headaches and symptoms including pain, nausea, vomiting and sensitivity to light and noise.

Black cohosh is a natural sedative for people who suffer from chronic anxiety, stress, insomnia or non-restful sleep.

Sleep

Sleep deprivation can make you feel fatigued, anxious and irritable at the best of times. As if sleep wasn't already important enough, it's also critical for hormonal balance. There are a number of hormones that are only secreted by the body at night. These include growth hormone, which is important for children's development as well as cell repair; prolactin, which promotes breast milk production; and oxytocin, which helps us to bond with our children and partners. These hormones are secreted by the pituitary gland, which influences the secretion of various hormones throughout the body and which is in turn influenced by how much sleep you get.

The stress hormone cortisol is also affected by sleep. Normally, cortisol levels should decrease throughout the day and be low in the evening when you go to sleep. Sleep disruption causes an increase in night-time cortisol. This in turn can affect insulin levels and potentially contribute to disorders related to that hormone, including insulin resistance and diabetes.

The good news is that the deleterious effects of sleep-induced hormonal imbalance are reversed when you start getting a good night's sleep. If you are suffering from hormone imbalance and are not getting an adequate quantity or quality of sleep, then this is one of the first things you should address.

In addition, as our modern lifestyle is very confusing for the brain and hormone production, you can also take some practical steps to support yourself.

- Make your bedroom your sanctuary; only use your bed for sleep, relaxation and sex.
- Keep the bedroom dark and cool.
- Try to go to bed at the same time every night, and wake up at the same time.
- Stop using smartphones and screens at least two hours before sleep (the blue light can disrupt melatonin production, which in turn affects getting to sleep and the various sleep cycles).
- Avoid caffeine after 1 p.m.

This list is not exhaustive, and many tips can be found online or with your GP; these are just ones that I've personally found to be very useful in my practice.

Exercise

Like so many other lifestyle factors, exercise can have a profound effect on your hormones.

The best-known effect of exercise is the release of endorphins, which can trigger feelings of intense satisfaction. In addition to releasing endorphins, exercise also increases blood levels of the hormone testosterone. This effect is more pronounced in men but can help to maintain bone and muscle strength in both sexes.

In addition to hormones, exercise can affect the neurotransmitters in your brain. Dopamine levels in the brain are increased after exercise. Dopamine can decrease stress levels and feelings of depression and promote a sensation of well-being. Serotonin is another hormone released when we do physical activity. This feel-good hormone promotes sleep, enhances mood and improve memory. If you're not getting any exercise, try to start small. Every little bit helps, and a consistent routine of even low-intensity exercise such as walking can have a positive impact on your hormones.

Gut health

Although there is an obvious physical distance between the gut and the mind, they are actually very close. This relationship has been extensively studied in recent years and understanding its ins and outs will hopefully help us to better nurture our gut and mind.

The key player in this gut-mind relationship is the community of microbes who live in our gastrointestinal tract. This population of microbes is known as the gut microbiota. Collectively they help to digest food, synthesise vitamins, fight infections, and, as discovered more recently regulate brain health. One of the first evidences of this gut-mind relationship (also called the gut-brain axis) came from a study where researchers showed that it was possible to transmit different behavioural traits between mice by transplanting their gut microbiota. Mice with a 'shy' personality would adopt a more 'adventurous' behaviour when carrying the gut microbiota from mice with an adventurous personality.[1] In humans, a trial has shown that administration of probiotics (live beneficial microorganisms) to patients with depression significantly improved their symptoms, particularly anxiety.

The messenger between the gut and the brain is the 'happy' chemical serotonin. Serotonin is well known for its role in regulating mood, appetite and sleep. The gut microbiota can affect levels of chemicals (or neurotransmitters – molecules that facilitate neuron communication in the brain). Certain types of microbes in the gut can directly stimulate the production and release of serotonin in the cells lining the colon. In fact these serotonin-producing cells account for more than 90 per cent of serotonin production in humans![2] No wonder these little organisms in your gut can have such a great influence on the brain and therefore on mood. If your gut isn't functioning correctly it may be that these cells aren't able to produce the right levels of serotonin needed to balance your mood.

Since it is becoming clearer that the community of microbes living in the gut can largely affect our outlook in life, it is crucial to take good care of these 'good guys'. Here are a few tips:

Replace

Eat foods rich in probiotics such as kefir, sauerkraut, kimchi, live yogurt and kombucha to build a strong army of good microbes.

---

1   Bercik, P., Denou, E., Collins, J., Jackson, W., Lu, J., Jury, J., . . . Collins, S. M. (2011). The intestinal microbiota affect central levels of brain-derived neurotropic factor and behavior in mice. *Gastroenterology*.
2   https://www.medicalnewstoday.com/articles/292693.php

Avoid

Avoid foods such as sugar, processed foods, excess gluten as well as alcohol. If you can't avoid these altogether, find a way to reduce intake and balance them with gut balancing foods.[3]

Avoid the overuse of antibiotics and painkillers; antibiotics can create a gut microbiota imbalance by killing good bacteria and painkillers can damage the gut lining.

Investigate

Check if you are suffering from any food reaction or food-related inflammation. Ongoing food reactions can trigger inflammation by leading to the production of inflammatory molecules called cytokines. Inflammation and cytokines damage the gut lining which leads to intestinal permeability. There is now evidence that inflammation is linked to depression.

If you often experience digestive symptoms, it may be helpful to perform a functional test that analyses your gut microbiota profile and can rule out a bacteria imbalance or infection (such as pathogenic bacteria or parasites).

Replenish

Replenish with supplements which can help to support your gut health and which include probiotics to replenish good bacteria, L-glutamine to reduce intestinal permeability and turmeric to reduce inflammation.

---

3   See https://www.mariongluckclinic.com/blog/gut-balancing-foods.html for more guidance on this.

Stress

Stress has a huge impact on our hormones and health. We are hard-wired to react to stress or what our body perceives to be danger. Today we are no longer under threat from predators and aggressors, but our daily life is far from being stress free and our body responds accordingly.

The stress response is released by the hypothalamus and prompts our adrenal gland to release the stress hormones adrenaline and cortisol. As a response, adrenaline will increase our heart rate and elevate blood pressure. Cortisol will also be released, increasing blood sugar in the bloodstream, while at the same time decreasing functions that are not immediately necessary in a fight-or-flight situation such as digestion and reproduction.

Chronic stress can expose us to persistent high levels of cortisol and adrenaline and may put us at risk of suffering from depression, anxiety, poor sleep, heart disease and weight gain. This should hopefully convince you that reducing stress is a worthwhile, if not essential, part of your hormone-balancing journey.

There are any number of options for reducing stress, including meditation, yoga, mindfulness, exercise and finding a hobby.

Yoga, meditation and mindfulness enhance neurotransmitters such as GABA, dopamine and serotonin, and lower cortisol levels. Yoga has been well known throughout the centuries as a positive anti-stress and life-affirming activity. Scientific studies have proven that it lowers cortisol levels in patients who are suffering from stress or depression.

Mindfulness and meditation calm the body and mind.[4] An increase in calming neurotransmitters like GABA is triggered during meditation. We know how important neurotransmitters are in the brain as they play a role in regulating anxiety and behaviour. They are increased when all is well, and decreased when we are stressed or depressed or in fight-or-flight mode.

What you decide to do to reduce your stress levels is less important than how consistent you are in doing it. Try to find a method or activity that you can stick to, and build a habit and routine around it.

How to speak to your GP about hormones

For many women, one of the hardest things about hormone imbalance is getting their doctor to take their concerns seriously. Unfortunately, most primary care physicians do not receive in-depth training in how to treat hormone imbalance. Therefore it is sometimes necessary for patients to help educate their doctors, or at least to point them in the right direction. Luckily, I find that most GPs are open-minded and keen to expand their knowledge, especially if it is in the service of helping one of their patients.

When visiting your GP, try to be well prepared and well informed. But don't go in looking for a fight. You and your GP should work as a team, and that requires a foundation of mutual respect.

You can begin the consultation by describing the symptoms you are experiencing and making it clear how they are affecting your

---

4   D. Krishnakumar et al., 'Meditation and Yoga can Modulate Brain Mechanisms that Affect Behavior and Anxiety – A Modern Scientific Perspective', *Ancient Science*, April 2015, 2(1), 13–19. Available at https://www.ncbi.nlm.nih.gov/pmc/articles/PMC4769029/.

well-being. If you have a hormone symptom diary, bring it with you. This will not only allow your GP to get a better understanding of the frequency and nature of your symptoms, but it also demonstrates your commitment to addressing the issue.

As a next step, explain that you believe your symptoms may be related to your hormones. It is important to do this in the correct way. These days doctors are (rightly) more sceptical about patients self-diagnosing with the help of 'Dr Google', and they may take you less seriously if you position your hormone issues as if they were a foregone conclusion. Instead, invite the doctor to investigate this possibility together with you.

If your GP seems receptive, you can show them the following questionnaire. It allows you to tick off the symptoms you have been experiencing and might point to a specific hormone imbalance. This is by no means a diagnostic tool; proper assessment requires an examination of symptoms as well as blood tests. But I find it can be a useful way to start the conversation about your potential hormone imbalance.

Oestrogen

- ☐ Hot flushes
- ☐ Night sweats
- ☐ Headaches
- ☐ Heart palpitations
- ☐ Dry skin
- ☐ Wrinkled skin
- ☐ Vaginal dryness
- ☐ Incontinence
- ☐ Poor memory
- ☐ Low energy
- ☐ Insomnia

Progesterone

- ☐ Heavy and painful periods
- ☐ Breast pain
- ☐ PMS
- ☐ Headaches
- ☐ Bloating
- ☐ Fluid retention
- ☐ Insomnia
- ☐ Depression
- ☐ Anxiety
- ☐ Mood swings
- ☐ Irritability

Testosterone

- ☐ Joint pain
- ☐ Loss of muscle tone
- ☐ Weight gain
- ☐ Low libido
- ☐ Low self-esteem
- ☐ Low energy

The first thing you should always ask from your GP is a female hormone blood profile. This is a blood test that will look at hormone levels in your bloodstream. Unfortunately, in recent years, under NICE guidelines, the NHS has removed hormone testing for women over the age of forty-five.

Your GP may not wish to carry out the blood test, or might argue that the results are meaningless because hormone levels constantly fluctuate. It is true that your hormones rise and fall significantly over the course of your cycle – that's why it's important to know what day of your cycle you are on when the blood is taken. Blood testing is also very important as it helps to understand what type of fluctuation you are experiencing. Is your oestrogen too high or too low; is your progesterone too high or too low; are your hormones balanced? The hormone symptom questionnaire opposite will help you and your doctor define what you are going through.

If your GP wants to prescribe you HRT, inform them that you only want to take bio-identical or body-identical hormones (as NHS doctors more commonly refer to them). Bio-identical hormones are licensed in the UK and are available on the NHS, but sadly many doctors are not aware of this.

If your doctor tells you there is no proof that personalised bio-identical hormone regimes are safer or better than synthetic alternatives, your best bet is to try to convince them on the basis of scientific evidence. At the end of this chapter there is a recommend reading section (see page 241), including a link to our website where you can print out a list of scientific papers and references that you can take with you to your doctor. This will allow them to assess the evidence and form their own opinion.

If your doctor wants to prescribe you antidepressants for your symptoms and this is not what you wanted or expected, you should remind them that you are not depressed and that you believe other treatments may be more appropriate.

Finally, in the extreme and hopefully very rare case in which your GP is wholly uncooperative, it may be time to seek a second opinion. You can try to see a different GP at your local NHS practice, or seek treatment privately. Luckily, there are many more doctors trained in and practising BHRT privately in the UK than ever before. Most of them will be found in London, but there are increasingly more options in other towns and cities across the UK.

Maintaining a hormone diary

Memory is a fickle thing, and with the chronic but episodic nature of many hormone imbalance symptoms it can be difficult at times to objectively characterise the severity and frequency of what you are experiencing. Often at the height of your symptoms it may feel as if they are a constant presence in your life, while during a lull you may feel yourself completely healthy, even symptom free. All too often we tolerate and normalise recurrent symptoms. They are easy to forget after they have resolved themselves, and we tend to ignore them until they return – at which point we regret very much not doing something about them.

A hormone diary is a good way to start mastering your hormones, and I often recommend my patients do this for at least three to six months. After a few months of noting your symptoms, you may be aware of certain patterns appearing – beyond the obvious ones you've been taught to look for. You may experience certain unexpected symptoms on certain days in the month with surprising regularity. These patterns will help both you and your doctor build a clearer picture of your hormonal health. As a bonus, it may help you to plan some aspects of your life to minimise the impact of your symptoms.

So what symptoms should you track? You can use the lists below as a starting point. Each of these symptoms may be a sign of hormonal imbalance, especially if they are recurrent. We all know that we have fluctuating hormones, and that it's normal to experience some degree of recurrent symptoms. The idea here is to capture those symptoms whose severity goes over and above what we consider normal. And I strongly believe that it should not be considered normal that our hormones make us feel miserable.

I've grouped the symptoms into those that are physical and those that are psychological in nature, but do not be surprised if you experience a mix of both.

Psychological	Physical
mood swings	cramps
insomnia	headaches
depression	bloating
low libido	breast tenderness
irritability	skin breakout
anger	heavy bleeding
food cravings	aching muscles
forgetfulness	low energy

There is no right or wrong way to record your symptoms in a diary, but I recommend a simple table like the example below. Recording a symptom on a specific day should be as straightforward as ticking a box; the result is easy to use to identify patterns. You can make things more complex by adding a scale for the severity of your symptoms, or notes to capture observations, but I believe it's best to keep things simple.

Day of the month	1	2	3	4	5	6	7	8	9	10	11	12	13	14
Period flow									X	X	X	X	X	
Period pain								X	X	X				
Aching muscles						X	X	X						
Digestive complaints														
Bloating							X	X	X	X				
Dizziness														
Headaches											X	X		
Mood swings				X	X	X	X	X						
Low energy									X	X				

The symptom diary is also something handy to take with you when you see your doctor. It will help them understand your symptoms and together you may spot patterns that point to a specific hormone imbalance. You also don't know how you will be feeling the day of your appointment, and so without a clear record of your symptoms you may be in danger of over- or understating their severity.

Hormone disrupters: how to protect yourself during pregnancy

We've recently seen increasing awareness and attention given to the prevalence and effects of hormone disrupters, and any lifestyle intervention should include limiting exposure to them to the greatest extent practical. Women who are pregnant and those with children should take particular care to protect themselves and loved ones from the effects of hormone disrupters.

The importance of protecting oneself from toxins and pollutants when pregnant should not come as a surprise to the reader. Babies *in utero* are constantly developing and growing. Foetal cells are taking in nutrients from the mother to utilise and build vital structures such as their immune, nervous and reproductive systems. They are building bones, muscles and all vital organs. The foetus will absorb whatever it is exposed to, be it nutrients or toxins.

Scientific studies have proven that chemicals in certain personal care products can pass through the placenta into the umbilical cord and thus into the foetal circulation. Our skin is a defence barrier against the majority of chemicals and toxins we encounter on a daily basis in our environment. However, skin products and lotions are formulated in such a way that they can be absorbed through the skin. These chemicals can also pose a risk during breastfeeding through the mother's milk.

We have been aware for a long time of the effects of certain foods and which ones to avoid during pregnancy. Sadly, we know much less about the effects of ingredients in personal care products, and this is where many potential hormone disrupters reside. Our understanding of how hormone disrupters affect pregnant women and babies is still evolving, but it would seem sensible to avoid these substances. Below are some chemicals you should watch out for in personal care products, especially when pregnant.

Phthalates are commonly found in perfumes, most scented products and nail polish, and worryingly in children's toys and children's care products. Phthalates are particularly dangerous to pregnant women and babies since they pose risks to the development of the reproductive system, brain and other organs.

Parabens are preservatives used to prevent the growth of mould and bacteria in cosmetics. They are very commonly used, so make sure to keep an eye out for paraben-free cosmetics and moisturisers.

Triclosan is actually a pesticide, but is used as an antibacterial agent in hand soaps and body wash. It is also a known hormone disrupter.

Topical sprays such as insect repellents or sunscreen pose a unique threat due to their potential for being accidentally inhaled. Once inhaled, chemicals in the spray can be easily absorbed into the bloodstream via the lungs.

The above advice doesn't just apply to pregnant women. While the effects of hormone disrupter exposure are particularly troubling for pregnant women, avoiding them at any stage in life is advisable.

Men's hormones – what you need to know

By now you probably feel like you're an expert on women's hormones. But it's possible that many of you have a male partner, and in that case, what about his hormones? Believe it or not, hormones and their change over time play an equally important role in men's lives as they do in women's.

The male version of the menopause is called andropause. Most men go through it without every really understanding what is happening to them. If your male partner begins to experience more frequent mood swings, irritability, headaches, stress, low libido, increased pain, increased abdominal fat or starts developing 'man boobs', chances are it's related to his hormones. Often the challenge with men is to get them to recognise the problem as something that a doctor could help with. Too often they will simply write it off as the effect of stress or too much work and try to carry on. However, if any of the above symptoms arise without a good explanation, your partner should be encouraged to have his testosterone and thyroid levels checked.

Hormones and antidepressants

Women are twice as likely as men to be on antidepressants. I have already written about this sad statistic and why the female gender is a frequent criterion for depression. We know that fluctuating hormones are one of the main reasons why women experience mood problems, and therefore we should always consider the possibility that a case of depression is caused by hormone imbalance.

However, for many people antidepressants can be a lifesaver, helping them to feel normal again and to cope with the various stressors in their lives. I would never advise someone to stop antidepressants when starting hormone replacement therapy. If their symptoms improve as a result of the HRT, it is still up to the patient and their regular GP as to whether they should continue on the same treatment and dose.

But there is a troubling tendency in some parts of the medical community to use antidepressants as a catch-all treatment for any mood-related issues. Depression can have many causes and we have now learnt how important it is to differentiate between them and treat patients accordingly. Antidepressants may help you to feel better, but they may also mask symptoms you should be paying attention to. And you should never, ever just take antidepressants and believe that everything is sorted.

Good health is all about maintenance, be it psychological, physical or hormonal. Continue to question, observe and challenge yourself and your doctor if you feel the antidepressant medication is not right for you. You can live without antidepressants, but your hormones are an integral part of your body and you're stuck with them for life.

Selected lifestyle protocols

This chapter so far has been about the many things you can and should do in support of your hormone health, but it's probably not realistic to do all of these things. In my years of helping patients recover through hormone replacement and lifestyle interventions I have developed a number of protocols designed to address specific hormone complaints. Think of these as your lifestyle intervention 'cheat sheets'. Find the protocols for the issues that bother you most and build a lifestyle intervention plan from them. As in all things, consistency is key. Try to create a realistic plan that you can stick to rather than a perfect plan. Start with small changes and build your way up. And of course, consider speaking to your doctor about hormone replacement therapy if you feel you could benefit from it.

PMS protocol

Nutrient	Dosage
vitamin B6	50–100mg per day
magnesium	200–600mg per day
L-methionine	500–1000mg per day (not with food)
L-theanine	200–600mg per day
omega-3	1000–3000mg per day
omega-6	500–1000mg per day

Increase consumption	Reduce or avoid consumption
complex carbohydrates	sugar
vegetables	caffeine
fruit	alcohol
nuts	processed foods
oily fish	refined carbohydrates
whole grains	trans/hydrogenated fats
purified water	

Lifestyle
minimise exposure to environmental hormone disrupters such as plastics
avoid smoking
use stress management techniques to reduce stress
increase exercise

Anxiety protocol

Nutrient	Dosage
magnesium	200–600mg per day
flaxseed oil	2–10g per day
rhodiola extract	250–750mg per day
L-theanine	50–600mg per day

How to Help Yourself

Increase consumption	Reduce or avoid
complex carbohydrates	alcohol
vegetables, especially dark leafy greens	caffeine
fruit	sugar
nuts and seeds	refined carbohydrates
oily fish	allergens
whole grains	

Lifestyle
eat regularly and never rush meals
do regular gentle exercise
avoid stressful situations if possible
use stress management techniques such as meditation and breathing
avoid recreational drugs

Perimenopause protocol

Nutrient	Dosage
vitamin B6	50–100mg per day
vitamin B12	1000–2000mcg per day
folic acid	800mcg per day
magnesium	200–600mg per day
L-theanine	200–600mg per day
omega-3	1000–3000mg per day
omega -6	500–1000mg per day
vitamin D3	2000IU per day

Increase consumption	Reduce or avoid
complex carbohydrates	alcohol
vegetables, especially dark leafy greens	caffeine
fruit	carbonated soft drinks
nuts and seeds	sugar
oily fish	trans/hydrogenated fats
whole grains	red meat
water	refined carbohydrates

Lifestyle
minimise exposure to environmental toxins
employ stress management techniques
do regular exercise

Sleep protocol

Nutrient	Dosage
B-complex	as per manufacturer's directions
5-HTP	50–300mg before sleep
magnesium	200–400mg before sleep
calcium	400–600mg before sleep
L-theanine	300–600mg per day

Increase consumption	Decrease or avoid
complex carbohydrates	alcohol
vegetables, especially dark leafy greens	caffeine
fruit	sugar
nuts and seeds	refined carbohydrates
whole grains	

Lifestyle
take regular gentle exercise
minimise stress
practise relaxation techniques as part of bedtime routine
promote balanced blood sugar, as low sugar levels can trigger early waking

Anxiety and low energy protocol

Nutrient	Dosage
magnesium	400mg at night
flaxseed oil	2–10g per day
rhodiola extract	250–750mg per day
L-theanine	50–600mg per day
chromium picolinate	200–600mcg per day
B-complex	as per manufacturer's instruction

Increase consumption	Decrease or avoid
vegetables, especially dark leafy greens	alcohol
fruit	caffeine
nuts and seeds	sugar
oily fish	refined carbohydrates
whole grains	allergens
complex carbohydrates	

Lifestyle
eat regularly and never rush meals
do regular gentle exercise
avoid stressful situations if possible
use stress management techniques such as meditation and breathing
avoid recreational drugs

Menopause protocol

Nutrient	Dosage
vitamin E	200–400IU per day
omega-3	1000–2000mg per day
vitamin D3	2000IU per day
black cohosh	200–400mg per day
dong quai	150–450mg per day

Increase consumption	Decrease or avoid
whole grains	alcohol
vegetables, especially dark leafy greens	caffeine
complex carbohydrates	sugar and salt
fruit	processed foods
nuts and seeds	trans fats
oily fish	red meat

Lifestyle
minimise exposure to stress
do regular gentle exercise
minimise exposure to environmental toxins

Thyroid support protocol

Nutrient	Dosage
selenium	200–400mcg per day
L-tyrosine	500–1000mg per day
iodine	150–450mcg per day
omega-3	1000–4000mg per day
zinc	15–30mcg per day
Vitamins A, C, E plus B-complex	1 tablet twice daily

How to Help Yourself

Increase consumption	Decrease or avoid
complex carbohydrates	brassica foods
vegetables	broccoli, Brussels sprouts, cabbage
fruit	pine nuts
nuts and seeds	soya beans
oily fish	turnips
whole grains	saturated and trans fats

Lifestyle
take regular gentle exercise
minimise exposure to stress
minimise exposure to environmental toxins

Adrenal support protocol

Nutrient	Dosage
Siberian ginseng	300–900mg per day
rhodiola extract	250–750mg per day
magnesium	200–600mg per day
vitamin C	1000–3000mg per day
zinc	15–30mcg per day
L-tyrosine	500–1000mg per day

Increase consumption	Decrease or avoid
complex carbohydrates	sugar
vegetables	refined carbohydrates
fruit	alcohol
nuts and seeds	caffeine
oily fish	salt
whole grains	saturated and trans fats

Lifestyle
take regular gentle exercise
minimise exposure to stress
minimise exposure to environmental toxins
avoid recreational drugs

Conclusion

In this modern day we are expected to be and do more than ever before, and finding our own balance is the only way we can really survive and thrive. It is no wonder that one in four people suffers from mental illness. As you have seen throughout this book, your hormones constitute every aspect of your well-being, and this final chapter has brought together all the nutritional and lifestyle factors to empower you to take charge and live at your optimum health.

Remember, it's not in your head; it can be your hormones, and it's a very real experience. I feel privileged to have helped so many women who felt they were losing their minds, and I hope this book will be useful in guiding you and your loved ones through the many phases of your lives.

Hormones really are your best friend.

RECOMMENDED READING

● ● ● ●

Hormones

Dr Marion Gluck, *It Must Be My Hormones: A practical guide to re-balancing your body and getting your life back on track*, Michael Joseph, London, 2017 (new edition).

Uzzi Reiss and Yfat Reiss Gendell, *The Natural Superwoman: The scientifically backed program for feeling great, looking younger, and enjoying amazing energy at any age*, Avery Publishing Group, New York, 2008.

Patrick Holford and Kate Neil, *Balance Your Hormones: The simple drug-free way to solve women's health problems*, Piatkus, London, 2011.

John Lee, *Natural Progesterone: The multiple roles of a remarkable hormone* (2nd edition), Jon Carpenter, Norton, 1999.

Nutrition

Magdalena Wszelaki, *Cooking for Hormone Balance: A proven, practical program with over 125 easy, delicious recipes to boost energy and mood, lower inflammation, gain strength, and restore a healthy weight*, HarperOne, San Francisco, 2018.

Dr Michael Ruscio, *Healthy Gut, Healthy You: The personalized plan to transform your health from the inside out*, The Ruscio Institute LLC, Walnut Creek, CA, 2018.

General well-being and relaxation

Fearne Cotton, *Calm: Working through life's daily stresses to find a peaceful centre*, Orion Spring, London, 2017.

Andy Puddicombe, *The Headspace Guide to . . . Mindfulness & Meditation: 10 minutes can make all the difference*, Hodder Paperbacks, London, 2012.

Matthew Walker, *Why We Sleep: The New Science of Sleep and Dreams*, Allen Lane, London, 2017.

INDEX

Index

Index

Index

Index

ABOUT THE AUTHOR

• • • •

Dr Marion Gluck trained as a medical doctor in Hamburg and has worked all over the world as a women's health specialist. She has been recognised as one of the top private doctors in the world for her pioneering treatment of hormonal imbalances using natural bio-identical hormones.

With over thirty-five years of medical practice, it was when she worked in Australia twenty years ago that she became aware of the increasing need for bio-identical hormones, and how every person should have both knowledge and access to them. Dr Gluck then founded the first UK clinic dedicated to bio-identical hormone replacement therapy, as a cutting-edge service that delivers personalised care and proven science to thousands of patients.

Dr Gluck is passionate about the potential of bio-identical hormones to change the lives of women and men for the better. It is her life's work to educate and promote their life-changing effects, with the aim of never hearing another story of suffering that could have been avoided.